PITUITARY AND PARAPITUITARY TUMOURS

Volume 6 in the Series

Major Problems in Neurology

JOHN N. WALTON, TD, MD, DSc, FRCP
Consulting Editor

OTHER MONOGRAPHS IN THE SERIES

PUBLISHED
Barnett, Foster and Hudgson: **Syringomyelia,** *1973*
Dubowitz and Brooke: **Muscle Biopsy: A Modern Approach,** *1973*
Pallis and Lewis: **The Neurology of Gastrointestinal Disease,** *1974*
Hutchinson and Acheson: **Strokes,** *1975*
Gubbay: **The Clumsy Child,** *1975*

FORTHCOMING
Behan and Currie: **Neuroimmunology**
Cartlidge and Shaw: **Head Injury**
Newsom Davis and Cameron: **The Neurology of Breathing and its Disorders**

Pituitary and
Parapituitary Tumours

JOHN HANKINSON, MB, BS, FRCS

Professor of Neurosurgery, University of Newcastle upon Tyne;
Consultant Neurosurgeon, Newcastle General Hospital and
Royal Victoria Infirmary, Newcastle upon Tyne.

M. BANNA, LRCP, MRCS, FRCR, MD, FRCP (Can.)

Associate Professor of Radiology, McMaster University
Medical Centre, Hamilton, Ontario, Canada.

With contributions by

A. L. CROMBIE, MB, ChB, FRCS(Ed.)
Consultant Ophthalmologist, Royal Victoria Infirmary,
Newcastle upon Tyne.

D. C. EVERED, MD, BSc, MRCP
Consultant Physician, Royal Victoria Infirmary,
Newcastle upon Tyne.

W. M. ROSS, MD, FRCS, FRCR
Consultant Radiotherapist, Newcastle General Hospital,
Newcastle upon Tyne

1976

W. B. Saunders Company Ltd   London · Philadelphia · Toronto

W. B. Saunders Company Ltd: 1 St. Anne's Road
Eastbourne, East Sussex BN21 3UN

West Washington Square
Philadelphia, PA 19105

833 Oxford Street
Toronto, Ontario M8Z 5T9

Library of Congress Cataloging in Publication Data

Hankinson, J
   Pituitary and parapituitary tumours.

   Includes index.
   1. Pituitary body—Tumours. I. el Banna, Mohamed, joint author
II. Title. [DNLM: 1. Pituitary neoplasms. WK585 H241p]
RC280.P5H36   616.9'92'47   76-24953
ISBN 0-7216-4495-3

Printed at W & J Mackay Limited, Chatham, Kent.

Print Number: 9 8 7 6 5 4 3

Foreword

Professor John Hankinson, Dr Mohamed Banna and their collaborators have written an excellent monograph on tumours arising in, or in relation to, the pituitary fossa. After a scholarly historical introduction, they discuss the general clinical presentation and pathology of these neoplasms and then separate chapters are devoted to pathophysiology, including tests of endocrine function, neuro-ophthalmology, radiology, surgery and radiotherapy. Each of the chapters included in this comprehensive monograph is an essay in its own right and, as a result, the reader will find here and there evidence of some duplication, but only sufficient to stress the importance of the topic under consideration in a somewhat different context. I know many readers will share my view that it is particularly useful to look at these tumours from the varying standpoints of an endocrinologist, an ophthalmologist, a surgeon and a radiotherapist. As a result of this multifocal approach, this survey is topical and comprehensive and gives a broad conspectus of current opinion concerning the diagnosis and management of these troublesome lesions. The chapter on pathophysiology underlines the explosive developments which have taken place in the last few years in endocrinology and the impact that these have had upon the management of pituitary lesions. Similarly, the neuro-ophthalmological approach underlines many new techniques of clinical assessment and investigation, and the chapter on radiology, illustrated by a large number of superb radiographs, clearly demonstrates the remarkable development of neuroradiology as a clinical science. But in the end the treatment of patients comes down to the important question as to whether the appropriate management is surgical, with or without endocrine replacement therapy and, if so, by what route. Should radiotherapy be given preoperatively or postoperatively and, if so, what technique is likely to be appropriate? These are questions which Professor Hankinson and Mr Ross consider logically and dispassionately with no evidence of conscious bias towards one method or the other.

Physicians and surgeons often disagree about the appropriate management of an individual patient, but the authors of this monograph have collected an admirable team of contributors from the Newcastle upon Tyne centre, each of whom has been prepared to consider these lesions in the light of results achieved in his own personal experience. This, in my opinion, is a comprehensive, valuable and enlightening monograph and I feel sure that many readers, whether they be neurologists, endocrinologists, neurosurgeons, neuroradiologists, radiotherapists or ophthalmologists, will share my view; it is a book which is likely to appeal to a very wide medical audience.

Newcastle upon Tyne, 1976   John N. Walton

Preface

Although it has many potential disadvantages, multiple authorship is justified in some subject fields, and in none more so than the consideration of the pituitary and its functions in health and disease. To present an account in any useful depth of the physiology and pathology of the medical, surgical and radiological problems to which the pituitary gives rise requires a team of experienced specialists, as indeed does their practical management. It has been our endeavour, therefore, to deal with these topics in sufficient detail for an understanding of the basic principles and at the same time to suggest a logical scheme of management. We are conscious of the numerous contemporary advances in the study of pituitary function, investigation and treatment and thus on leaving the press some of our statements may be open to challenge; nevertheless, we hope that while some of those interested in the pituitary will know more than we have expressed in some particular sections of the book, all will find some enlightenment in others.

We wish to thank our colleagues who have allowed us access to cases which are referred to in the text. The craniopharyngioma series was collected from a number of hospitals and acknowledgements have been made in previous publications. The illustrations in the radiology section are for the most part from the Regional Neurological Centre, Newcastle upon Tyne and the Medical Centre of McMaster University, Hamilton, Ontario; we are most grateful to Dr Gordon Gryspeerdt and Dr Arnold Appleby of the former institute and to Dr W. P. Cockshott of the latter. The illustrations in the pathology section are partly from the National Hospital for Nervous Diseases, Queen Square, through the help of Professor William Blackwood, and partly from Newcastle upon Tyne by courtesy of Professor B. E. Tomlinson. All the illustrations of computerised tomography are from Hamilton General Hospital, Ontario, Canada. Reference is made in individual captions to many authors and publishers who supplied us with material of their own. To all of them we wish to extend our gratitude.

Dr P. S. Ramani, now in Bombay, gave us valuable assistance in a detailed review of 221 cases of pituitary adenoma treated in Newcastle and we wish to thank him. We have had skilled and cheerful secretarial assistance from Mrs Anne Storey, Mrs Eileen Matthews and Miss Laurie MacKenzie. It is a pleasure to acknowledge the encouragement and advice given by Professor John N. Walton, the Consulting Editor of this series of monographs and the help and patience of Mr William R. Schmitt of the W. B. Saunders Company.

Newcastle upon Tyne, England   John Hankinson
Hamilton, Ontario   Mohamed Banna
1976

Contents

CHAPTER ONE

Terminology, Embryology and Anatomy

M. BANNA

TERMINOLOGY

The word pituitary is derived from the Latin word 'pituita' meaning mucous secretion or phlegm, which in turn came from the Greek 'ptuo', to spit (Wain, 1958). Aristotle spoke of pituita secreted from the brain as a part of the cooling process which he thought was a function of the brain. This view was also shared by Galen (c.A.D. 130–200). The gland was first described in 1524 by the Italian anatomist Berengarius. Andreas Vesalius (1514–64) called it 'glandula pituitam cerebri excipiens' and stated that it was the source of mucus secreted into the nose. Franciscus Sylvius (1614–72) and Raymond Vieussens (1641–1716) considered that the structure played a part in the elaboration of cerebrospinal fluid, a viewpoint also expressed by Thomas Willis in 1664. The notion of mucus secretion was finally disposed of by Schneider in 1672 but the term pituitary persisted.

The word hypophysis is derived from the Greek for 'lying under' which describes the gland's anatomical position under the brain. Infundibulum was the term used by Rufus of Ephesus for a funnel-shaped passage and has since been applied to various structures. Vesalius used infundibulum as an alternative term for the attachment of the pituitary gland to the brain.

According to the *Encyclopaedia Britannica*, Richard Lower, in 1672 was probably the first to ascribe an 'endocrine' role to the gland, for he considered that it removed fluid from the cerebrospinal fluid and secreted it into the blood stream. However it was not until 1840 that Mohr described obesity associated with pituitary tumours (Skinner, 1961). A disease associated with hypertrophy of the hands, feet and face – acromegaly – was first noted by Saucerotte in 1772 and later by Alibert (1822), Magendie (1839) and Sir Samuel Wilkes in 1869. It was first clearly defined by the French neurologist, Pierre Marie in 1886. In an *Essay on Acromegaly* he wrote: 'There exists an affection characterised chiefly by hypertrophy of the feet, hands and face, which I propose to call "acromegaly", that is to say, hypertrophy of the extremities.' In 1887 Minkowski called attention to the constancy of the pituitary enlargement in this disease.

The description of two types of epithelial cells (chromophil and chromophobe) is usually credited to Flesch (1884), although they had previously been mentioned by Hannover in 1844. The first proper description of a chromophobe adenoma is uncertain, but much of the descriptive histology of pituitary tumours is attributed to Benda (1900).

In 1904 Erdheim, a Viennese pathologist, discovered by accident a few islets of

1

squamous epithelial cells in the hypophyseal region which he believed were remnants of Rathke's pouch. He noted that there was a close similarity of these cells to the epithelial content of some suprasellar tumours and suggested that both tumour and islets had the same origin. The former he identified as a separate group, which he named 'hypophyseal duct neoplasm'. This term remained in use until 1932 when Cushing introduced the term 'craniopharyngioma' to describe the tumour discovered earlier by Erdheim. The word craniopharyngioma was much easier to use and despite the fact that it is less accurate, because Rathke's pouch is an evagination from the oral cavity and not the pharynx, it has been universally accepted and continues to be widely used.

EMBRYOLOGY

The pituitary gland consists of two main parts; an epithelial portion derived from Rathke's pouch and giving rise to the anterior lobe, and a neural segment developing from the floor of the diencephalon and forming the posterior lobe.

Rathke's pouch can first be identified when the embryo is 3 mm in length at about the third week of intra-uterine life. It appears as a distinct shallow recess in the roof of the stomodeum just in front of the oropharyngeal membrane (Figure 1.1). The pouch

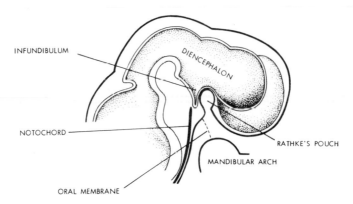

Figure 1.1. Schematic sagittal section of the head of the embryo to show the anatomical position of Rathke's pouch.

gradually deepens and extends towards the floor of that portion of the neural plate destined to be the diencephalon. Its caudal end then narrows, becoming a hollow stalk known as the craniopharyngeal duct which remains patent until about the 17-mm stage. Subsequently, it is transformed into a solid core of cells known as the epithelial stalk (Figure 1.2). As the mesoderm forming the skull base develops, most of the cells forming the epithelial core disappear but some may remain until adult life as ectopic pituitary remnants (Figure 1.3). These may persist within the sella but outside the capsule of the gland (hypophysis accessoria cranii), within the body of the sphenoid bone (hypophysis accessoria cranio-

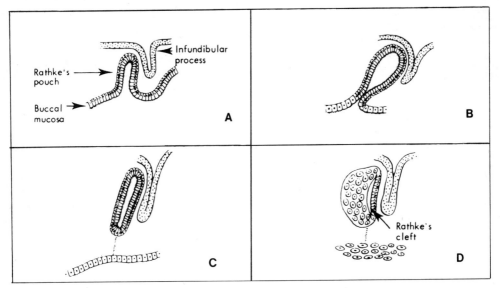

Figure 1.2. Diagrammatic sketch of the development of the hypophysis cerebri. A. Evagination of oral mucosa to form Rathke's pouch. B. Closure of the buccal end of Rathke's pouch and transformation of the cephalic end into a vesicle. C. The vesicle remains connected to the buccal mucosa by an epithelial stalk which gradually disappears but remnants of cells resulting in ectopic anterior lobe tissue may remain along its track. D. The rate of cell multiplication varies in different parts of the vesicle being faster in the anterior wall which forms the pars distalis and slower in the posterior wall which becomes the pars intermedia.

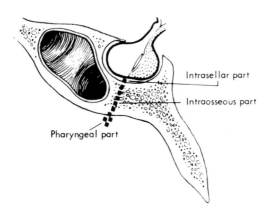

Figure 1.3. Ectopic anterior lobe tissue is shown in solid black squares.

pharyngei) or in the posterior wall of the pharynx (hypophysis accessoria pharyngei). The latter may be large enough to be considered as an accessory hypophysis.

While the cells forming the caudal end of Rathke's pouch gradually disappear, the cells constituting the cephalic end (now a vesicle) proliferate to form the anterior lobe of the pituitary gland. The rate of cellular multiplication varies in different sites of the vesicle but is fastest in the anterior wall giving rise to the pars distalis. The cells of the posterior wall which are very slow in growth give rise to the pars intermedia. The original cavity of the vesicle thus diminishes in volume and forms Rathke's cleft which occasionally remains until adult life as a small cyst. From the anterolateral angles of the hypophyseal evagination two small epithelial ridges develop. They grow upwards and fuse in front of the pituitary infundibulum forming the pars tuberalis, so called because of its relation to the tuber cinereum.

The mechanism by which the pituitary fetal cells are differentiated into chromophobe, eosinophil and basophil cells is not known. There are two main concepts, unitarian and dualistic. The unitarians propose that the three types of cells are merely different functional stages in the cycle of a single cell; the chromophobes starting the cycle and the basophils terminating it as degenerating cells. Others believe that the chromophobes are formed from either the basophil or the eosinophil cells by amitotic nuclear division followed by clearing of the cytoplasm around one of the daughter nuclei. The dualists, on the other hand, maintain that the chromophobes and the chromophils are two completely different types of cells, each having a separate origin. A third view, which is now the most widely accepted, suggests that these cells are interchangeable. The chromophils and the basophils can arise from the chromophobes by elaboration of specific granules but they can also revert to chromophobes by a process of degranulation.

ANATOMY

The anterior lobe of the pituitary gland (pars anterior or adenohypophysis) consists of the pars distalis, the pars tuberalis and the pars intermedia (Figure 1.4). It forms the main bulk of the gland and is somewhat kidney-shaped, its concavity being directed backwards and embracing the posterior lobe. These two lobes are separated from each other by

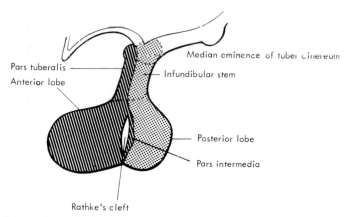

Figure 1.4. Hatched area: Parts developing from Rathke's pouch. Dotted area: Parts developing from the floor of the diencephalon.

Rathke's cleft. The posterior wall of the cleft is formed by the intermediate lobe (pars intermedia). This consists of a thin, poorly vascularised layer of finely granular basophil cells between which are masses of colloid material.

The pars posterior (the neurohypophysis or pars nervosa) is attached to the diencephalon by the infundibulum of the pituitary gland which is directed downwards and forwards and contains a funnel-shaped recess from the cavity of the third ventricle (the infundibular recess). The infundibulum is surrounded by the pars tuberalis.

In adults the pituitary gland weighs approximately 500 mg. It is oval or spherical in shape, its antero-posterior diameter being the longest. On average the gland measures approximately 12.5 mm in antero-posterior diameter, 11.5 mm in transverse diameter and 6 mm in vertical diameter. The gland is lodged within the sella turcica (Latin: turkish saddle) which forms the roof of the sphenoidal air sinus. Between the sinus and the glandular elements of the gland there are the capsule of the gland, a fibrovascular layer of connective tissue, and the lamina dura of the floor of the sella. The diaphragma sellae is a double fold of dura mater covering the pituitary fossa which is pierced by the infundibulum. The dural orifice for the pituitary infundibulum varies in size; it may be narrow just allowing the pituitary stalk to pass through, or it may be widely open allowing the arachnoid membrane of the suprasellar cistern to herniate into the sella.

Histologically the anterior lobe is formed of three main types of cells which differ from each other in their staining properties. Some stain deeply with eosin and are termed eosinophils (acidophilic or alpha cells). Others stain with basic dyes and are termed basophilic (cyanophils or beta cells). The third type of cells take up very little stain and are called chromophobe cells. The ratio of these types varies with age and sex and in the same individual the number of cells may vary with the increased demand of pituitary hormones as for example during pregnancy. In addition to the main cell types, the anterior pituitary lobe may contain a few transitional cells having a faint polychromatic stain, some fetal or undifferentiated cells and minute vesicles containing colloid material. The fetal cells are more often seen in the periphery of the lobe whereas the eosinophils are more condensed in the central part. The chromophobes and basophils lie in between these two zones. The pars nervosa is composed almost entirely of fusiform and irregularly shaped cells which are provided with delicate processes named pituicytes.

CLINICAL ANATOMY OF THE PITUITARY GLAND

An accurate knowledge of the anatomical relationships of the pituitary gland is essential to an understanding of the clinical manifestations of the various pathological lesions in the area. Since visual failure is an exceedingly common manifestation, the optic pathways should be considered first.

The optic chiasm has an antero-posterior diameter which varies from 4 to 13 mm, a transverse diameter of 10 to 20 mm and its thickness varies from 3 to 5 mm (Walsh and Hoyt, 1969). The optic nerves diverge forward from the chiasm at an acute angle which varies from one individual to another depending on the distance between the optic foramina and the length of the optic nerves. The distance between the medial walls of the optic foramina varies from 20 to 11.5 mm and the intracranial portion of the optic nerves may be 6 to 21 mm in length (Bull, 1956).

It must be emphasised that in the majority of cases the optic chiasm lies posterior to the sulcus chiasmaticus (sulcus interopticus) and not above it as the name implies (Figure 1.5). The position of the chiasm can be determined at pneumoencephalography by the point of chiasmatic insertion – the notch between the optic and infundibular recesses at the anterior end of the third ventricle (Bull, 1956). In 90 per cent of cases the optic chiasm lies partially or totally above the diaphragma sellae. In about 5 per cent the chiasm lies above the sulcus interopticus (pre-fixed chiasm) and in another 5 per cent the chiasm lies on and behind the dorsum sellae (post-fixed chiasm). These individual variations in the position of the optic chiasm are partly responsible for the fact that identical lesions may produce different visual manifestations. The chiasm is separated from the diaphragma sellae by the suprasellar

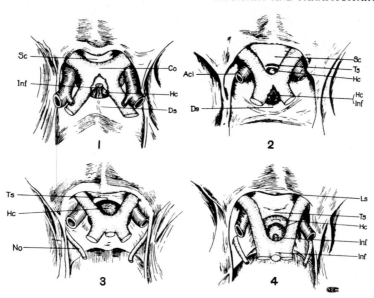

Figure 1.5. The location of the optic chiasm in relation to the sulcus chiasmaticus (after Schaeffer, 1924).

1. Optic chiasm located in part on the chiasmatic sulcus, the remaining portion resting upon the diaphragma sellae. This type was found in 5 per cent of the bodies examined.

2. Optic chiasm wholly located over the diaphragma sellae. This type was found in 12 per cent of the bodies examined.

3. Optic chiasm also wholly located over the diaphragma sellae, a small portion projecting on to the dorsum sellae. This type was found in 79 per cent of the bodies examined.

4. Optic chiasm located on and behind the dorsum sellae. This type was found in 4 per cent of the bodies examined. Sc = sulcus chiasmatis; Inf = infundibulum; Co = chiasma opticum; Hc = hypophysis cerebri; Ds = dorsum sellae; Aci = arteria carot. int.; Ts = tuberculum sellae; No = nervus oculomotorius; Ls = limbus sphenoidalis.

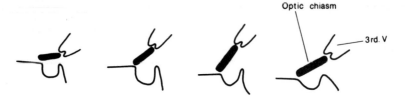

Figure 1.6. This diagram illustrates variation between different individuals in the degree of tilting of the optic nerve and chiasm. (After Bull, 1956)

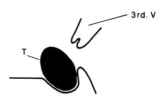

Figure 1.7. Forward tilting of the sella combined with a post-fixed chiasm may, on very rare occasions, allow a pituitary tumour to grow between the optic nerves in front of the chiasm with little or no visual impairment and absence of deformation of the third ventricle. (After Bull, 1956)

cistern which varies in depth from 3 to 10 mm. This implies that a suprasellar tumour less than one centimetre in diameter which may be totally asymptomatic in one patient may produce significant visual disturbance in another.

Other anatomical variations influencing the symptomatology of pituitary and parapituitary tumours include the tilt of the plane of the optic nerves (Figure 1.6), and the tilt of the sella (Bull, 1956). When there is an unusual degree of forward tilting of the sella combined with a long intracranial portion of the optic nerves, a tumour theoretically may grow in front of the chiasm between the two optic nerves, producing only minor degrees of visual impairment (Figure 1.7). However, it is generally recognised that the visual symptoms produced by pituitary tumours are not only the result of mechanical compression of the chiasm but are, perhaps more significantly, due to interference with its blood supply. Much depends on the anatomy of the circle of Willis; for instance, compression of a hypoplastic anterior cerebral artery on one side may be of less significance than compression of the larger artery on the opposite side.

The vessels supplying the optic chiasm (Dawson, 1958; Bergland and Ray, 1969) can be divided into three groups (Figure 1.8):

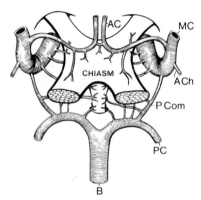

Figure 1.8. Diagrammatic illustration of the arterial supply of the optic chiasm. AC = Anterior cerebral artery which gives rise to the superior chiasmal arteries supplying the superior surface of the chiasm. MC = Middle cerebral artery. Proximally several small arterial branches (superior hypophyseal arteries) are seen arising from the carotid siphon. P Com = Posterior communicating artery. PC = Posterior cerebral artery. A Ch = Anterior choroidal artery.

1. *Superior chiasmal arteries*. These are derived mainly from the horizontal segment of the anterior cerebral arteries and vary in number from one to four vessels on each side. They join with small branches from the ophthalmic and internal carotid arteries to form a prechiasmal arterial anastomosis occupying the angle between the optic nerves; the anastomosis is occasionally supplemented by a small twig from the anterior communicating artery.
2. *Inferior chiasmal arteries*. Small branches from the superior hypophyseal arteries supplying the chiasm from below.
3. *Arteries supplying the central decussating fibres of the chiasm*. The central part of the chiasm, including its superior and inferior surfaces, receives its blood supply from the vessels in the second group. Some of these vessels penetrate and traverse the thickness of the chiasm to supply its superior surface.

Interference with the blood supply of the visual tract leads to a variety of disturbances, from complete optic atrophy to a small field defect depending on the distribution of the artery involved. If the chiasm is elevated by a suprasellar neoplasm the vessels most distorted are those supplying the decussating fibres; hence the preponderance of bitemporal field defects in these cases.

The optic chiasm is, of course, involved by the upward growth of pituitary tumours and further extension in this direction, in addition to interference with the hypothalamic–pituitary connections, may compress the foramen of Monro and produce hydrocephalus. Tumour extension in a lateral direction distorts the structures within the cavernous sinus (Figures 1.9 and 1.10). These include the carotid artery surrounded by a

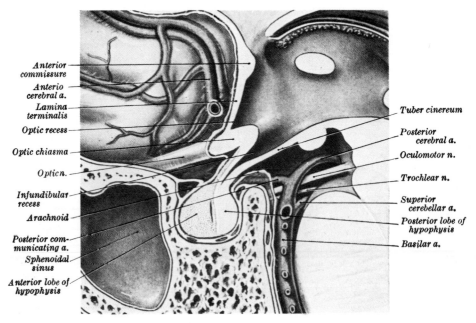

Figure 1.9. Sagittal section through the hypophysis (semidiagram from Gray's *Anatomy*). Note in particular the proximity of the optic chiasm to the contents of the sella.

plexus of sympathetic nerves, the abducent nerve inferolateral to the artery and the oculomotor, the trochlear, the ophthalmic and the maxillary divisions of the trigeminal nerve on the lateral wall of the sinus. Tumour extension into the sphenoidal sinus is common but it very rarely leads to leakage of cerebrospinal fluid. This is because inferiorly 'the capsule' of the pituitary gland blends with the meninges and neither can be identified as a separate structure. Tumours extending in a posterior direction, having destroyed the dorsum sellae, may present as a posterior fossa neoplasm and in such cases the facial nerve may be involved.

These are the directions of tumour growth which are commonly encountered but there are a few patients with massive pituitary tumours, particularly craniopharyngiomas, in which the tumour may extend into the frontal lobes, the thalamus, the temporal lobes or even down the clivus into the cervical canal. This type of lesion is rare and almost always confined to children.

The Blood Supply of the Hypophysis Cerebri

There is a voluminous literature on the arterial supply of the pituitary gland. Of the most recent publications Powell, Baker and Laws (1974) and Pribram, Boulter and McCormick

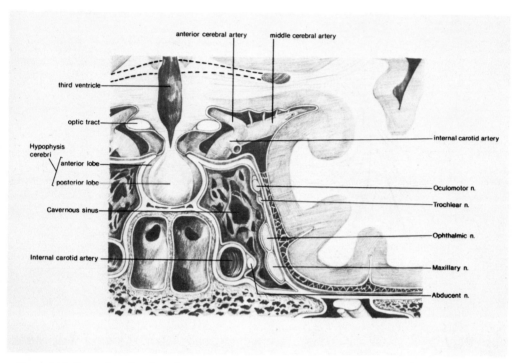

Figure 1.10. Coronal section through the middle cranial fossa to show the relation of the hypophysis to the structures within the cavernous sinus (semidiagrammatic).

(1966) may serve as key references to previous work.The following paragraph is quoted from the paper by Pribram, Boulter and McCormick (1966), but it should be pointed out that the vessels described are seldom seen in a conventional angiogram. They may be rendered visible more frequently, particularly in children, by magnification angiographic techniques.

'The arterial blood supply of the hypophysis is derived from the inferior and superior hypophyseal arteries which arise from the carotid siphon (Figure 1.11). The inferior hypophyseal artery supplies the posterior lobe while the superior hypophyseal artery supplies the anterior lobe. The inferior hypophyseal artery arises from a common trunk which takes origin at the junction of the proximal vertical and horizontal segments of the cavernous internal carotid artery. The trunk from which it arises may be termed the meningo-hypophyseal trunk since it distributes 3 branches which supply the hypophysis and the meninges. The branches are, respectively : the inferior hypophyseal artery, the dorsal meningeal artery, and the tentorial artery. The inferior hypophyseal artery passes upwards and medially to reach the lateral surface of the posterior lobe of the hypophysis where it divides into superior and inferior divisions and anastomoses with similar branches from the other side. The dorsal meningeal artery passes behind the dorsum sellae to ramify on the posterior surface of the clivus, and then anastomoses with similar branches from the contralateral internal carotid artery. The tentorial artery passes backwards within the edge

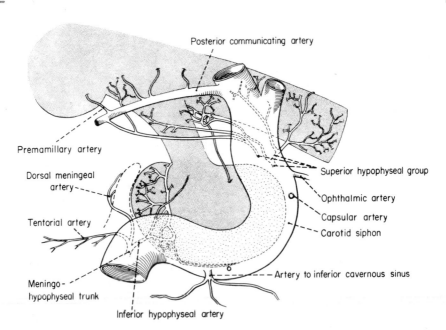

Figure 1.11. Arterial supply of the hypophysis cerebri. Upper carotid siphon and posterior communicating artery have been elevated to reveal the pituitary stalk. (Reproduced from Powell et al (1974) and credited to McConnell, 1953)

of the tentorium. It also anastomoses with its fellow from the opposite internal carotid artery. There is considerable variation in the origin of these vessels. Thus, while one may be able to demonstrate a classic meningo-hypophyseal trunk on one side, the various branches may arise individually on the opposite side. The superior hypophyseal arteries arise from the postero-medial aspect of the internal carotid artery shortly after it emerges from the cavernous sinus. The arteries run upwards and medially to supply the optic nerve, the optic chiasm, and the anterior lobe of the hypophysis.'

The blood circulation within the hypophysis cerebri differs from any other part of the brain in that it has two capillary beds and blood sinusoids similar to those in the liver. Hence, this type of circulation is referred to as the hypophyseal portal system (Xuereb, Prichard and Daniel, 1954). Springing from the superior and inferior hypophyseal arteries are numerous ascending and descending branches which encircle the hypophyseal stalk

(Figure 1.12). These infundibular arteries run a somewhat tortuous course before penetrating the neural tissue to break up into capillaries (first capillary network), which drain through efferent vessels into hypophyseal portal vessels. Each hypophyseal portal vessel breaks up within the pars distalis into a number of sinusoidal channels (Figure 1.13). The sinusoids anastomose freely with one another and thus form a dense network (the second capillary bed). They drain through small collecting channels of variable size into the venous sinuses surrounding the pituitary body.The hypophyseal portal vessels are the only efferent blood vessels to the epithelial tissue of the pars distalis, which has no direct blood supply (Xuereb, Prichard and Daniel, 1954).

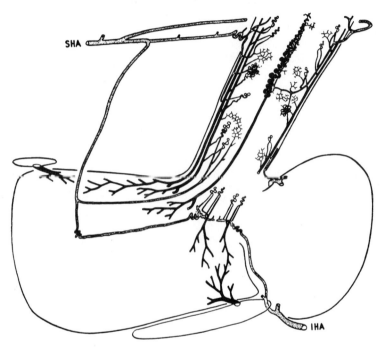

Figure 1.12. Diagram to show the vessels of the hypophyseal portal system. The various types of capillary formations in the hypophyseal stalk and lower infundibular stem constitute a first capillary bed. This extensive capillary system drains through long or short hypophyseal portal vessels into the sinusoids of the pars distalis, the second capillary bed. From the sinusoids blood is drained through collecting veins into the venous sinuses which surround the pituitary body. The first capillary bed is supplied chiefly by the superior hypophyseal artery (SHA), but the lower infundibular stem receives in addition some arterial blood from the inferior hypophyseal artery (IHA). (By courtesy of Professor P. M. Daniel and the editor of the *Quarterly Journal of Experimental Physiology.*)

REFERENCES

Bayoumi, M. L. (1947) *Pathological Study of Pituitary Tumours Especially as Regards the Types, Incidence and Course.* MD Thesis, Edinburgh.

Benda, C. (1900) Beitrage Zur normalen, und pathologischen Histologie der menschlichen Hypophysis Cerebri. *Archiv fur Anatomie und Physiologie* (phys. Abstract), **cccxiv**, 373.

Bergland, R. & Ray, B. S. (1969) The arterial supply of the human optic chiasm. *Journal of Neurosurgery*, **31**, 327–334.

Bull, J. (1956) The normal variations in the position of the optic recess of the third ventricle. *Acta Radiologica*, **46**, 72–80.

Cushing, H. (1932) The craniopharyngiomas. In *Intracranial Tumours.* pp. 93–98. London: Bailliere, Tindall and Cox.

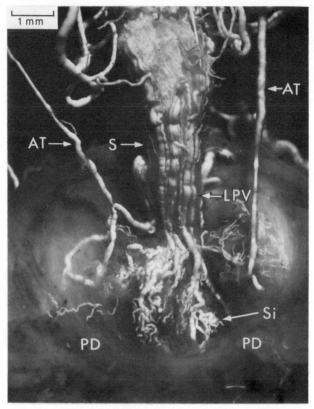

Figure 1.13. Human pituitary gland and stalk seen from in front and above. The vessels have been injected with neoprene latex and the tissues partly macerated, to show the long portal vessels (LPV) running down the stalk (S) and breaking up into the sinusoids (Si) of pars distalis (PD). AT, artery of the trabecula. (By courtesy of Professor P. M. Daniel)

Dawson, B. H. (1958) The blood vessels of the human optic chiasm and their relation to those of hypophysis and hypothalamus. *Brain,* **81,** 207–217.

Dott, N. M. & Bailey, P. (1925–26) A consideration of the hypophyseal adenomata. *British Journal of Surgery,* **13,** 314–366.

Erdheim, J. (1904) Uber Hypophysenganggeschwulste und hirncholesteatome Sitzungsberichte der Mathematisch-Naturwissenschaftlichen Klasse der Kaiserlichen Akademie der Wissenschaften 113. *Abteilung,* **LLL,** 537–726.

Flesch, M. (1884) *Tageblat der 57 Naturforscher Versammlung* (Magd.). Quoted by Bayoumi (1947).

Marie, P. (1886) Sur deux cas d'acromegalie. *Revue de Medicine,* **6,** 297–333.

Powell, D. F., Baker, H. L. Jr & Laws, E. R. Jr (1974) The primary angiographic findings in pituitary adenomas. *Radiology,* **110,** 589–595.

Pribram, H. F. W., Boulter, T. R. & McCormick (1966) The roentgenology of the meningo-hypophyseal trunk. *American Journal of Roentgenology,* **98,** 583–594.

Skinner, H. A. (1961) *The Origin of Medical Terms.* 2nd edition, pp. 327, 328. Baltimore: Williams and Wilkins.

Wain, H. (1958) *The Story Behind the Word.* p. 249. Springfield, Illinois: Charles C. Thomas.

Walsh, F. B. & Hoyt, W. F. (1969) *Clinical Neuro-Ophthalmology,* 3rd edition. Baltimore: Williams and Wilkins.

Xuereb, G. P., Prichard, M. M. L. & Daniel, P. M. (1954) The hypophyseal portal system of vessels in man. *Quarterly Journal of Experimental Physiology,* **39,** 219–229.

CHAPTER TWO

Pathology and Clinical Manifestations

M. BANNA

CLASSIFICATION OF PITUITARY AND PARAPITUITARY TUMOURS

Using the word 'tumour' to mean a space-occupying lesion (tumere = to swell), tumours occurring in the pituitary and parapituitary region can be divided into two mains groups:

A. Neoplastic tumours
1. Pituitary adenoma
2. Craniopharyngioma
3. Meningioma
4. Optic nerve glioma
5. Hypothalamic glioma
6. Chordoma
7. Cholesteatoma
8. Germinoma or ectopic pinealoma
9. Hypothalamic hamartoma
10. Infundibuloma
11. Myoblastoma
12. Metastasis
13. Carcinoma of sphenoid sinus and nasopharynx
14. Tumours of the base of the skull

It should be noted in this group that cholesteatomas and hamartomas may be considered as congenital malformations rather than neoplasms.

B. Non-neoplastic tumours
1. Aneurysm
2. Sphenoidal air sinus mucocele
3. Dilated third ventricle
4. Arachnoid cysts
5. Granulomas
6. Pituitary abscess

Primary tumours of the skull base are beyond the scope of this book and of the non-neoplastic lesions, sphenoid sinus mucocele, dilated third ventricle and arachnoid cysts are discussed in the radiology section, Chapter 5.

PITUITARY ADENOMA

Pituitary adenomas are benign tumours arising within the capsule of the pituitary gland. According to the cell origin of these tumours, three types are identified: (1) chromophobe adenoma, (2) eosinophil (acidophil or alpha cell) adenoma, (3) basophil (or beta cell) adenoma. To these should be added, (4) mixed tumours in which a varying proportion of eosinophils and, rarely, basophils are found among the chromophobe cells.

Chromophobe Adenoma

This is the commonest pituitary tumour in adults. The age distribution is shown in Figure 2.1. They are commonest in the third and fourth decade with a slight preponderance in males.

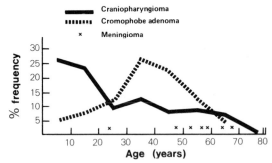

Figure 2.1. Age distribution among the three most common tumours in the pituitary and parapituitary region. It is based on a retrospective study of 60 pituitary adenomas and 7 suprasellar meningiomas from the Regional Neurological centres in addition to 160 craniopharyngiomas from various hospitals.

Macroscopic appearances

A chromophobe adenoma arises within the capsule of the pituitary gland in the pituitary fossa, which is thereby usually enlarged. Massive pituitary lesions may extend in one or more of the following directions (Blackwood, 1965):
1. Through the aperture in the diaphragma sellae pressing upon the inferior surface of the optic chiasm, first producing upper temporal field defects. Sometimes the optic nerve is pressed against a pulsating anterior cerebral artery producing a lower field defect.
2. Downwards into the sphenoidal air sinus.
3. Upwards between the frontal lobes.
4. The tumour may splay and displace the anterior part of the third ventricle, but obstruction of the foramen of Monro leading to an obstructive hydrocephalus is uncommon.
5. It may grow upwards and forwards surrounding the terminal portions of the internal carotid arteries, or laterally into the tissue bordering the Sylvian fissure.
6. The tumour may enlarge into the cavernous sinus involving cranial nerves III, IV, V and VI and, rarely, may cause obstruction of the internal carotid artery.
   The tumour is usually soft and depending on its vascularity, it may be greyish or maroon-

pink in colour. It may undergo cystic degeneration, but more important is the liability to spontaneous haemorrhage within these tumours leading to the syndrome of pituitary apoplexy. A large adenoma remaining within its capsule is often described as 'massive adenoma' (Figure 2.2). The term 'invasive adenoma' refers to a tumour which bursts out of its capsule.

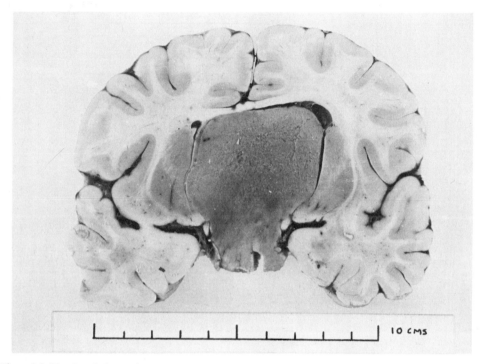

Figure 2.2. Massive pituitary adenoma. Note the presence of a distinct line of cleavage between the tumour and the surrounding brain in spite of the enormous size of the tumour.

Histological appearances (Figure 2.3)

Three main types have been recognised:
1. The diffuse type. This is composed of masses or sheets of pale rounded or polygonal cells with central spheroidal nuclei, intersected by a delicate connective tissue stroma. The tumour cells vary considerably in size, not only in different tumours, but also in different parts of the same tumour.
2. Sinusoidal or papillary type. The tumour cells are elongated and arranged around the supporting blood vessels.
3. Mixed type, where both the diffuse and sinusoidal patterns are present within the same tumour, is common.

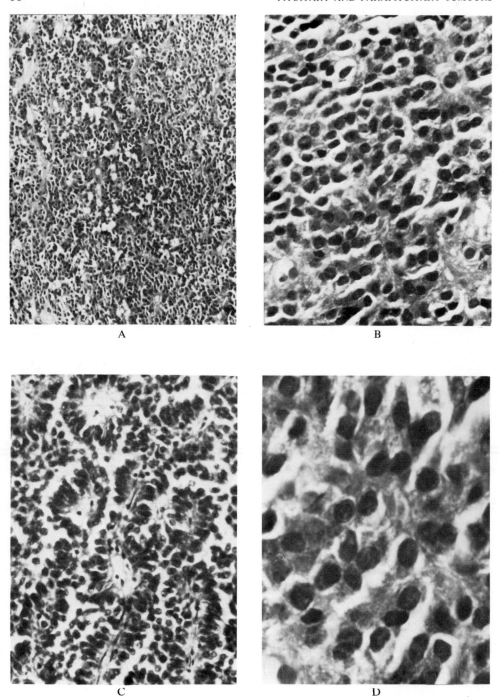

Figure 2.3. Histology of chromophobe adenoma. A. Note hypervascularity and the tendency of tumour cells to perivascular arrangement (x 125). B. Diffuse type of chromophobe adenoma composed of masses or sheets of polygonal cells (x 500). C. The sinusoidal type (x 300). D. Irregularity of the cell nuclei, as shown in this illustration, does not indicate malignant change in chromophobe adenoma (x 1000).

Clinical manifestations

Many chromophobe adenomas are neither entirely chromophobic nor functionless but contain a varying proportion of acidophilic or basophilic cells and either type may lead to some manifestations of the diseases related to them. A considerable proportion of chromophobe adenomas are also associated with increased prolactin levels in the blood. It is not certain whether this is due to autonomous secretion by the tumour or to interference with the production of one of the normal pituitary hormones, the presence of which inhibits lactation (Forbes et al, 1954). Nevertheless, the term chromophobe is generally used to describe a pituitary adenoma not associated with acromegaly or Cushing's syndrome. This type of lesion causes pressure atrophy of the normal pituitary gland and leads to a wide variety of clinical manifestations. Thus, the patient may present initially to the ophthalmologist, the gynaecologist, the general physician or the endocrinologist before he is referred to the neurologist or neurosurgeon. Patients, particularly in the older age group, may remain unaware of their illness until an enlarged pituitary fossa is discovered on skull radiographs taken for some other cause, and some small tumours may be detected for the first time at postmortem examination. There are also a few patients who present as an emergency with symptoms suggestive of meningeal irritation, subarachnoid haemorrhage or in coma from hypopituitarism. Bearing in mind this wide spectrum, the clinical manifestations of chromophobe adenoma will be discussed under the following headings. Some of these manifestations may, of course, be common to other pituitary neoplasms.

Headache. This is a common feature of all pituitary tumours and is generally thought to be due to stretching of the dura mater. It may subside when the sella has become widely distended and the diaphragm has ruptured. When headache persists, it is usually relieved by sellar decompression. A subtemporal decompression, on the other hand, which usually relieves the headache of other intracranial tumours, has no effect on pituitary headaches (Dott and Bailey, 1925). Dural distension alone may not explain the persistent headaches which sometimes accompany acromegaly, nor does it explain the headaches in those cases with a normal sella (Gordon, Hill and Ezrin, 1962). Thus, there may be some causes, other than capsular distension, leading to headache. According to A. L. Crombie (See Chapter 4) the incidence of headaches in the cases he personally examined was 55 per cent in acromegaly and 40 per cent in patients with chromophobe adenoma, the supraorbital region was the most common site followed by pain in or around the eyes. Dott and Bailey (1925) described the headache as typically a dull aching pain, or a sensation of pressure and discomfort, referred to one or both temples or behind the eyes. Occipital, frontal, temporal and generalised headaches have been described (Gordon, Hill and Ezrin, 1962) and it seems that there are no features characteristic of headaches from a pituitary tumour.

Headache due to ventricular obstruction is rare in cases of pituitary adenoma: In a personal review of 60 pneumoencephalograms of proven adenomas, only a few showed slight ventricular dilatation, and none showed obstructive hydrocephalus. The latter was much more common in craniopharyngioma and with invasive tumours. Evidence of increased intracranial tension leading to headache, vomiting and papilloedema is usually a terminal feature of hypophyseal disease. This may arise either as a result of the actual bulk of the intracranial protrusion or by virtue of complicating obstructive hydrocephalus (Dott and Bailey, 1925). Ventricular dilatation, on the other hand, from basal meningeal adhesions has been reported following surgery and irradiation of pituitary adenoma (Shenkin and Crowley, 1973).

Visual disturbances. This is dealt with extensively in Chapter 4. Suffice it here to mention that about 70 per cent of patients with chromophobe adenoma complain of blurred vision and that visual field defects may be seen in 95 per cent of such cases. Involvement of the third, fourth or sixth cranial nerves producing diplopia, strabismus or ophthalmoplegia is present in about 11 per cent (Sheline, Boldrey and Phillips, 1964). These high figures emphasise the importance of eye signs in pituitary disease.

Depression of sexual function. The first clinical manifestations of a chromophobe adenoma are often related to depletion of the gonadotrophic hormones. In women who are in the fertile age group, this is usually obvious and leads to irregular, scanty menstruation followed by amenorrhoea. Primary amenorrhoea due to pituitary adenoma is rare, but the author has investigated two cases referred from one infertility clinic within the space of a year.

In men, loss of libido is an early manifestation of pituitary adenoma, but the patient may not spontaneously complain of such symptoms. In late cases, oligospermia or azoospermia may be present associated with testicular atrophy.

Galactorrhoea. This is a common presenting feature of pituitary tumours, be they chromophobe adenomas or prolactin secreting micro-adenomas. Careful examination of the breasts with manual expression will often reveal breast secretion which has not been apparent to the patient. The combination of galactorrhoea, amenorrhoea and low urinary FSH is referred to as the Forbes–Albright syndrome (Forbes et al, 1954).

Changes in the skin and hair. In patients with hypopituitarism the skin is often thin, smooth, unduly dry and hairless. The axillary and pubic hair is scanty and the hair over the head may be fine and dry. Male patients do not need to shave as frequently as previously and in them the pubic hair may be of a feminine distribution.

Symptoms related to depletion of thyroid, adrenal and posterior pituitary hormones. These include generalised weakness, increased fatigability, cold intolerance and diabetes insipidus. Adrenocortical insufficiency (Addison's disease) secondary to a pituitary tumour is generally slow in onset leading to anorexia, episodes of nausea and vomiting, hypoglycaemia and, if severe, to hypotension and collapse.

The incidental chromophobe adenoma

Microscopic chromophobe adenomas are said to be the commonest intracranial lesion to be found incidentally at routine postmortem examination. In a series of 149 chromophobe adenomas, there were 29 patients (19.5 per cent) in whom the diagnosis had been unsuspected and was not made until necropsy. In 22 patients (15 per cent of the series) the tumour was of microscopic size and in 7 (4.5 per cent) the pituitary glands were enlarged. In none of these cases was death related to the pituitary adenoma (Sheline, Boldrey and Phillips, 1964).

Cystic chromophobe adenoma

Henderson (1939) reported that 17 per cent of the chromophobic adenomas and 6 per cent of eosinophilic ones are largely or entirely cystic. The fluid within the cyst may be dark red blood or xanthochromic fluid. Intrasellar cysts are usually unilocular, but those extending outside the sella are sometimes multilocular. The cyst wall consists of tumour tissue of varying thickness and the incidence of cyst formation does not appear to be influenced by previous radiation. The clinical manifestations of cystic tumours do not differ from those of the solid type.

Invasive Pituitary Adenoma

There is a very small number of chromophobe adenomas, probably 2 per cent to 3 per cent which has been designated by various authors as malignant chromophobe adenoma, adenocarcinoma or pituitary carcinoma (Dott, Bailey and Cushing, 1925; Henderson, 1939; Bailey and Cutler, 1940; Jefferson, 1940). Tumours labelled as such differ from the average chromophobe adenoma in many respects. They are usually massive. They have a shorter clinical history and are associated with symptoms other than those due to pressure on the pituitary gland or optic chiasm. To the naked eye, these tumours, perhaps because of their rapid growth, appear to burst out of their capsule and invade the adjacent structures. They may grow into the cavernous sinus and incorporate, rather than displace, the carotid artery and the cranial nerves. They may extend into the frontal or temporal lobes, or they may penetrate the sphenoid sinus and emerge into the nasopharynx. It has recently been suggested that invasive adenomas are more common in adolescents (Ortiz-Suarez and Erickson, 1975). On histological examination, cellular pleomorphism and mitosis are present in a greater number than the average adenoma, and to a number of pathologists these features indicate that some adenomas are at least locally malignant. Others object to the use of the word malignant and refer to these tumours as 'invasive'. Rubinstein (1972) stressed the fact that cellular pleomorphism and a few mitotic figures should not be equated with clinical malignancy. He stated that occasionally cells from a pituitary adenoma may disseminate into the cerebral sub-arachnoid space, but neither this event, nor the atypical cytological features, nor the occasional development of distinct subdural or sub-arachnoid nodules some distance from the main mass are sufficient in his view to warrant the diagnosis of a malignant tumour.

There are, however, very few chromophobe adenomas giving rise to extracranial metastases and all pathologists agree that such tumours should be labelled malignant. Thus, from a clinical point of view, three types of adenomas can be recognised: the average, the invasive and the malignant (Scholz, Gastineau and Harrison, 1962).

The clinical picture of invasive adenomas

As stated earlier, these tumours are usually massive. Their clinical manifestations are related to the direction of tumour growth which may be discussed under the following headings:

Hypothalamic extension. The outstanding features in these cases are somnolence, thirst, polyuria, obesity and temperature variation; hyperpyrexia was probably the cause of death in one of the cases described by Jefferson (1940).

Frontal extension. This may cause epilepsy, personality change or anosmia, due to involvement of the olfactory bulbs.

Temporal extension. Temporal lobe involvement may lead to epilepsy (including uncinate attacks), homonymous hemianopia and hemiparesis.

Extension into the cavernous sinus. Here the third and fourth cranial nerves are affected more frequently than the sixth, which lies on the outer side of the carotid artery and is protected by it. The fifth may be also involved, resulting in ptosis, diplopia, ophthalmoplegia and facial analgesia. Lateral extension into the cavernous sinus was considered by Jefferson (1940) as a definite indication of malignancy, but he pointed out that only slight pressure on the oculomotor nerve may be sufficient to cause diplopia. This alone does not necessarily indicate tumour extension into the cavernous sinus.

Nasopharyngeal extension. It should be pointed out that the spongy bone of a non-pneumatised sphenoid sinus is eroded more easily than the compact bone of a fully pneumatised one. Tumour extension into the sinus is also common, but protrusion into the posterior portion of the roof of the nasal cavity is exceedingly rare. Kay, Lees and Stout (1950) found only three cases among 192 adenomas and referred to two described earlier by Bailey and Cutler (1940). Henderson (1939) noted nasopharyngeal extension in eight of the 338 cases of Cushing's series. This type of tumour extension, when small, was not suspected clinically and was only detected at postmortem examination. Large extension was present in some patients at the time of their first hospital admission, and in one the presenting symptom was nasal obstruction from the tumour extension.

Cerebrospinal fluid rhinorrhoea from invasive pituitary adenomas

This is a rare complication of pituitary tumours, but pituitary tumours are the commonest cause of tumour-induced cerebrospinal fluid rhinorrhoea (Ommaya et al, 1968). It is more liable to occur in association with invasive lesions, either as a result of direct pressure atrophy of the roof of the sphenoid sinus or indirectly from ventricular obstruction. In the first case, there is escape of CSF through the posterior nasal space, but in the second, the high intracranial pressure leads to erosion of the cribriform plate of the ethmoid bone and escape of CSF into the anterior nasal space. Another rare complication which may follow upon direct invasion of the sphenoid sinus is spontaneous intracranial 'aerocele' or 'pneumatocele'. One such case has been reported in a 30-year-old man presenting with headaches and visual deterioration whose skull radiographs showed air within and about an enlarged pituitary fossa (Sage and McAllister, 1974).

Eosinophil Adenoma

These tumours seldom attain the massive size described in some of the chromophobe adenomas. More frequently, they remain confined to the pituitary fossa which becomes uniformly expanded. Occasionally, the tumour bulges above the sella and compresses the optic chiasm. Microscopically, the tumour cells can be differentiated from the chromophobe type by special stains.

Acromegaly

As stated in Chapter 1, acromegaly has been known since about the middle of the eighteenth century, and was fully described by Pierre Marie in 1886. Nevertheless, it was Cushing who in 1909 established the relationship of the disease to tumour formation or, in some cases, to hyperactivity of the pituitary eosinophilic cells. In his address to the sixtieth annual session of the American Medical Association he stated: 'When hypophyseal overactivity of the eosinophilic cells commences in youth, gigantism occurs; when in adult life, acromegaly; when commencing in youth and continuing into adult life, a combination of the two may be seen.'

Acromegaly, when advanced, can be diagnosed at a glance. The patient's coarse features, the prominent supra-orbital ridges, large bulbous nose, jutting lower jaw and thick lips are all well known. The hands and feet are large and spade-like: The patient has a slightly kyphotic posture and his voice is harsh, due to thickening of the vocal cords. Profuse sweating, often accompanied by a disagreeable odour may be a feature. On examination, there is hypertrophy of practically all the tissues. The skin is thick and oily and in some parts of the body, such as the palms of the hands and the scalp, it may be deeply corrugated, giving a very remarkable appearance on the scalp described by Cushing as 'the bull-dog scalp of acromegaly'. The jaw is protruding (prognathism), leading to malocclusion and wide spacing of the teeth. Visual field defects may be present (see Chapter 4) and hypertrophy of the internal organs (splanchnomegaly or visceromegaly) may be detectable on clinical examination. The osseous changes are evident and are dealt with in Chapter 5. All these manifestations follow an insidious course over 20 to 30 years or longer. They occur so gradually that usually the diagnosis is not made for several years and often comes to light by chance. Old photographs show a striking contrast with the patient's present appearance.

Table 2.1. The presenting symptoms in 164 patients with acromegaly.

Presenting symptoms	No.	Percentage	Frequency of symptoms
None	50	30.5	
Altered appearance	58	35.4	
Other	56	34.1	
headache			34 (20.7%)
carpal tunnel syndrome			6 (3.7%)
amenorrhoea			6 (3.7%)
fatigue			2 (1.2%)
pituitary failure			3 (1.8%)
deterioration of vision			6 (3.7%)
heart failure			3 (1.8%)
backache			1 (0.6%)
weight gain			1 (0.6%)

According to Houston, Joiner and Trounce (1972), early complaints are of easy tiredness, muscular aching, asthenia, excessive sweating and tingling in the fingers from median nerve compression (carpal-tunnel syndrome). Later, progressive enlargement of the hands and feet may be noticed, usually when buying gloves or shoes, or of the head when buying a hat. Enlargement of the jaws may cause dentures not to fit. Later symptoms are due to failure of gonadal function, amenorrhoea in women and loss of libido and impotence in men. However, gonadal symptoms were stated by Cushing to be a frequent early manifestation of the disease. In a recent study of 164 acromegalics, Alexander (1975) found that about one-third presented with a complaint of altered appearance, one-third were investigated following the casual observation of acromegalic features by general practitioners or in patients attending hospital for unrelated conditions, while the clinical presentation in the remaining third was directly or indirectly attributed to the complications of acromegaly. The presenting features in these patients are summarised in (Table 2.1). In another large series of 100 cases of acromegaly reported by Gordon et al (1962), the incidence of various clinical manifestations was: headaches 50 per cent, visual disturbances 40 per cent, irregular menstruation and amenorrhoea 33 per cent, generalised degenerative arthritis 30 per cent, decreased glucose tolerance 50 per cent, clinical diabetes mellitus 18 per cent, and of these latter cases, two were insulin resistant. High blood pressure exceeding 150/100 mm Hg was present in 18 patients, hyperparathyroidism in two, goitre in 24, hyperthyroidism in three and exophthalmos in six. Two patients complained of non-puerperal galactorrhoea, but seven women had successful pregnancies after the onset of acromegaly. The sella turcica was of normal size in 24 per cent, compared to 10 per cent on conventional radiography and 1.4 per cent on tomography in other series (McLachlan and Wright, 1970).

From a prognostic point of view, untreated cases of acromegaly are more liable to develop cardiovascular and cerebrovascular complications. This is because in them, the incidence of hypertension, atheroma, diabetes mellitus and cardiomyopathy are more common. Wright et al (1970) investigated the natural history of the disease in 55 dead acromegalics and concluded that the number of deaths was almost twice that expected in the general population of similar age and sex.

'Inactive' or 'burned-out' acromegaly. Although in the majority of cases acromegaly is a slowly progressive disease, the acromegalic process may occasionally become self-limiting, often by spontaneous infarction which may be associated with acute hypopituitarism and shock (Males and Townsend, 1972). In these patients, all the physical changes of acromegaly may be present without elevation of the plasma growth hormone levels. In one such case at pneumoencephalography there was a large suprasellar cistern extending into the sella and outlining a shrunken tumour within an enlarged pituitary fossa, an appearance similar to the 'empty sella' following surgery or irradiation of the pituitary gland. The patient, a young woman in her twenties with acromegalic features, gave no history of shock and her growth hormone levels were not elevated (Figure 2.4). Such

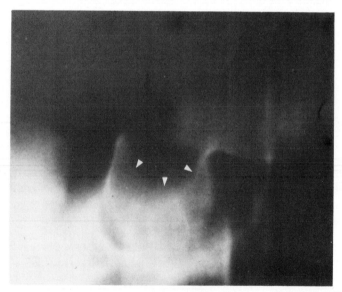

Figure 2.4. Burned-out acromegaly. Pneumoencephalo-tomogram showing a diaphragma sellae (arrow-heads) sunken into an enlarged pituitary fossa. Note the large suprasellar cistern.

radiographic appearances in untreated 'inactive' acromegaly must be very rare. Assessment of the activity of the disease depends solely on the estimation of growth levels in the blood (*British Medical Journal,* 1974).

Pituitary gigantism

According to the *Encyclopaedia Britannica,* the conventional definition of a giant is a height exceeding 200 cm in men and 187 cm in women. Pituitary gigantism resulting from excessive growth hormone secretion before closure of the long bone epiphyses is rare, there being only about 200 cases recorded in the literature. Human growth hormone does not promote growth of long bones by direct action on the epiphyses but acts through the intermediary of a second hormone formed in the liver and peripheral tissues and until recently known as sulphation factor because it promotes sulphate uptake by cartilage. It is now known as somatomedin (Ciba Review, January 1973).

Pituitary giants are of low sex drive and potency, but they may become local celebrities because of their enormous heights. Their life-span is not great and they usually die in early adult life if untreated. Description of pituitary gigantism is not complete without reference to Charles O'Brien, the famous Irish giant whose huge size was attributed in the eighteenth century to his conception on the top of a haystack. He was 249 cm in height and died at the age of 20 years. Reference was made in the Ciba Review (January, 1973) to a larger giant, Jan Van Albert, who measured 287 cm but unlike his predecessor his remains do not reside in the Royal College of Surgeons and his large pituitary fossa was not proven by Cushing himself. It has been said that had John Hunter opened the giant's skull in 1783, endocrinology might have had an earlier birth (Bergland, 1965).

Pituitary dwarfism

This is mentioned here, not for any relation with eosinophilic adenoma, but because it is the direct opposite of pituitary gigantism, the main abnormality being deficiency of the growth hormone. In about half the cases, the cause is unknown and is labelled as idiopathic. In about one-third, the condition occurs secondary to craniopharyngioma and in the remainder it is due to other lesions compressing or destroying the pituitary gland in early childhood.

Idiopathic pituitary dwarfism is a sporadic disease which is at least twice as common in males. The child is born of normal weight, has normal parents and siblings and begins to show signs of growth retardation at the age of one to three years. This sometimes remains unnoticed until he starts school, and he may reach only 125 to 150 cm in height in adulthood. Intelligence is normal and is farther advanced than physical development. The patient maintains the fine features of a child and can perhaps be best described as having the brain of an adult and the figure of a child. The condition is sometimes referred to as the Lorain–Levi syndrome and its characteristic features are:
1. Normal growth during the first one or two years of age.
2. Delayed skeletal maturity.
3. Sexual infantilism.
4. Normal intelligence.

Unlike the majority of cases of secondary pituitary dwarfism, there is no deficiency of the antidiuretic hormone, since the disease affects only the function of the anterior lobe (Brasel et al, 1965). The sella is normal but all the pituitary trophic hormones, compared to individuals of the same age, are diminished (Williams, 1968). On the basis of these endocrine and radiological abnormalities, differentiation from other types of dwarfism is seldom a problem (Bailey, 1973).

Basophil Adenoma

These are usually minute in size and seldom large enough to justify the term adenoma. They are often associated with bilateral adrenal hyperplasia and were originally thought to be the primary cause of Cushing's syndrome.

None of Harvey Cushing's voluminous contributions to medical literature have given rise to more controversy than the pathogenesis of the syndrome which now bears his name. This is because basophilic adenomas are almost invariably associated with hypertrophy of the adrenal cortex and because the clinical features of the syndrome may result from primary tumours of the adrenal gland and other lesions beyond the scope of this book (Binder and Hall, 1972).

Clinical manifestations of basophil adenoma

Giving the Harvey Society Lecture at the New York Academy of Medicine in 1933, Cushing selected two cases to illustrate the clinical manifestations of basophil adenoma. The first was that of a precocious adolescent girl, 10 years of age, who acquired a peculiar plethoric appearance with an abnormal growth of hair on brows, lips and chin. She became increasingly obese, with progressive increase of purplish striae atrophicae. She had persistent backache and became round-shouldered with a loss of four cm in measured stature, due to decalcification of the vertebrae. She had high blood pressure and her menses which had continued for three years suddenly ceased.

The second case was that of a 33-year-old woman, who at 19 years of age developed amenorrhoea, plethoric adiposity, purple striae atrophicae and hypertension. Relative subsidence of symptoms occurred for 10 years, followed by exacerbation, multiple fractures, glycosuria and hypertension. During the course of the disease she complained of headache, polydipsia, polyuria, palpitation, shortness of breath, generalised weakness and easy bruising. She showed hypertrichosis and hirsutism and suffered from a nervous breakdown in the later stages of her illness. At post mortem a pituitary basophil adenoma was present and both adrenal glands were enlarged. There were extensive atherosclerosis, chronic nephritis and nephrocalcinosis, hypertrophy of the cardiac musculature and generalised osteoporosis.

These two cases represent not only the classical manifestations of Cushing's syndrome, but also the complications that may arise. The disease is primarily a disorder of young adult life and it is at least four or five times more frequent in females. The common presenting features are amenorrhoea, obesity, hirsutism, hypertension and symptoms related to spinal osteoporosis. Other complaints may include generalised weakness, headaches, polyuria and polydipsia and personality changes may be noted. On examination there is abnormal distribution of fat involving the face and trunk but sparing the extremities. The patient is often described as having a plethoric appearance, a 'moon face', 'piggy eyes', a 'buffalo hump', a protruberant abdomen and looking like a 'lemon on toothpicks'. There is usually some degree of virilism and some patients may become heavily bearded. There are purple striae particularly over the abdomen, breast, thighs and axillae. Hypertension and oedema are frequent and diabetes mellitus not uncommon. Other clinical findings include excessive bleeding from simple wounds and scratches, polycythaemia rubra and electrolyte imbalance. Patients with Cushing's disease have a diminished inflammatory response and are more susceptible to infection. They also have increased secretion of hydrochloric acid and pepsinogen which predisposes to peptic ulceration and perforation. Bone marrow activity is increased in Cushing's disease leading to an increased red cell, platelet and neutrophil count but the lymphocyte and eosinophil counts are reduced.

The endocrinal disturbances that account for many of these clinical manifestations have been analysed by Nocenti (1968). The excess glucocorticoids have a major effect on carbohydrate, protein and fat metabolism. On carbohydrates they promote gluconeogenesis and interfere with peripheral glucose utilisation leading to diabetes mellitus. They have a definite catabolic effect on protein metabolism leading to muscular wasting, weight loss, thinning of the epidermis and osteoporosis. Fat is mobilised and redistributed on the face, suprascapular area and on the trunk, but not on the extremities. Cholesterol is deposited in the blood vessels, accounting for the extensive atheromatous changes. Due particularly to increased secretion of mineralocorticoids, there is sodium retention and potassium loss. The former leads to oedema and contributes to the development of hypertension. Hypokalaemia increases muscle weakness and probably plays a part in the development of polyuria. Calcium metabolism is also affected, resulting in hypercalcaemia, increased calcium excretion, osteoporosis and renal calculi. The withdrawal of protein components from the skin results in a thinning of certain areas to form broad, deep, purplish scars or striae. Thinning of the vessel walls results in increased vessel fragility, small capillary haemorrhages and delayed healing of wounds. Amenorrhoea, hirsutism and virilism are accounted for by excessive androgen secretion, while the high corticosteroid levels may predispose to the various psychiatric disturbances that are common in Cushing's syndrome.

Pituitary Apoplexy*

Among the unusual presentations of a pituitary tumour, the clinical syndrome known as pituitary apoplexy deserves special mention because it occurs probably more frequently than the approximately 120 instances reported in the literature would suggest. Its recognition is often delayed, and prompt treatment can sometimes reverse even the more severe neurological deficits.

The term 'pituitary apoplexy' (Bleibtreu, 1905) should be reserved for the dramatic clinical disturbance that follows the sudden enlargement of a pituitary adenoma. It should not describe the frequent operative or pathological finding of haemorrhage within an adenoma whose detection has been allowed by the development of the more gradual and classical syndrome of pituitary deficiency with chiasmal compression, neither should it describe the haemorrhage found in normal pituitary glands of patients succumbing to shock, sepsis or Sheehan's syndrome (Kraus, 1945; List, Williams and Balyeat, 1952; Locke and Tyler, 1961).

The word 'apoplexy' is ideally suited to this still rare presentation of a pituitary adenoma, for the sudden expansion of the tumour is a consequence of either haemorrhage into, or swelling from infarction of, the adenoma (Müller and Pia, 1953). The clinical states that follow such an enlargement result from an acute pituitary insufficiency and the compression of neighbouring structures (Kirschbaum and Chapman, 1948; Brougham, Heusner and Adams, 1950; Uihlein, Balfour and Donovan, 1957; Wright and Ojemann, 1965), the suddenness and severity of the syndrome depending upon the magnitude of the vascular insult.

While the diagnosis will readily come to mind when the syndrome develops in a patient with a known adenoma, difficulty is usually experienced when the disturbance occurs in a patient hitherto asymptomatic.

Anatomy

The sella turcica describes the profile of a mid-sagittal section of the sphenoid bone. While this time-honoured but fanciful reference to Turkish equestrianism reasonably describes the hypophyseal fossa of the dried skull, the in vivo arrangements are more elaborate. In the living state, the shallow depression in the body of the sphenoid bone is converted into a fossa

---

*The section on Pituitary Apoplexy was contributed by Andrew Talalla, Associate Professor of Surgery (Neurological), McMaster University, Canada.

of variable depth by the cavernous sinuses, each applied to the lateral aspects of the pituitary gland.

Unique among the dural venous sinuses, each cavernous sinus contains, in additon to a venous network or plexus, the internal carotid artery as well as the third, fourth and sixth cranial nerves and the two divisions of the trigeminus (Figure 2.5).

Above the pituitary fossa is the optic chiasm. The pituitary stalk leaves the pituitary fossa through a variable-sized aperture in the dural roof or diaphragm of the sella. The sub-arachnoid space, faithfully conforming to the contours of the anterior wall of the third ventricle and the posterior portions of the gyri recti, gains access to the pituitary fossa through this opening in the diaphragm and forms a collar of variable width about the upper pole of the pituitary gland.

Enlargement of the gland affects all the borders of the fossa, but with an explosive enlargement of the gland it is only the non-bony borders that can accommodate the sudden increase in volume. These accommodating borders are the diaphragm of the sella and the two cavernous sinuses, all of which are sensitive to stretch and all innervated by branches from the first division of the trigeminal nerve.

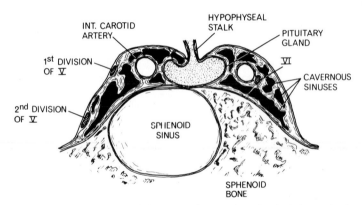

Figure 2.5. Coronal section through sphenoid bone showing relationship of pituitary gland to the structures within the cavernous sinuses.

Clinical syndromes

With an understanding of the aetiology of the sudden expansion of a pituitary adenoma and the derangements of anatomy that can follow it, various syndromes of pituitary apoplexy can now be appreciated.

Meningeal inflammation. The expulsion of necrotic or haemorrhagic adenomatous material into the sub-arachnoid space can cause an acute but sterile meningitis, a sub-arachnoid haemorrhage, or a blend of the two. Sudden, generalised and often severe headache with neck stiffness, fever and chills can be accompanied by a peripheral leucocytosis. The cerebrospinal fluid may show a pleocytosis or be uniformly, though lightly, blood-stained.

Acute visual loss. Compression of the anterior visual pathways is caused by the upward extension of the adenoma. The classical chiasmal syndrome of pituitary disease is often extended to cause unilateral and sometimes total blindness (Cairns, 1938; Weinberger, Adler and Grant, 1940; Shenkin, 1955; Meadows, 1968; Walsh and Hoyt, 1969).

Cavernous sinus syndromes. All or part of a unilateral or bilateral ophthalmoplegia with ptosis can occur abruptly. When bilateral, it is rarely symmetrical. When unilateral and partial, it is said to affect the abducens earliest or most severely. Extensive encroachments upon the cavernous sinus can affect the first division of the trigeminal nerve, the second division being spared because, running lower down, it is protected by the sphenoid bone which here forms the medial border of the cavernous sinus.

Head pains. An abrupt onset of severe anterior head pain without symptoms or signs of meningeal irritation is probably caused by the sudden stretching of the diaphragm of the sella which is innervated by meningeal branches of the first division of the trigeminal nerve. Unilateral, predominantly eye pain is a consequence of distension of the walls of the cavernous sinus in a parasellar expansion. The pain is a referred phenomenon affecting structures innervated by the ophthalmic division of the trigeminal nerve. The unilateral pain often accompanies, but can sometimes precede, the development of a cavernous sinus syndrome.

Acute stroke. Perhaps the rarest of the varied manifestations of pituitary apoplexy is the sudden total occlusion of the internal carotid artery in its intracavernous course, a consequence of a lateral expansion of an adenoma affecting almost certainly a diseased artery (Schnitker and Lehnert, 1952; Jolley and Mabon, 1958; Adriano and Al-Mondhiry, 1967).

The commonplace is a variable blend of all but the last of these syndromes, so that the pattern of disturbances presented to a puzzled clinician is usually one of an acute illness with meningeal irritation and the more focal neurological abnormalities related to the rate and direction of the expansion – hypopituitarism, ophthalmoplegia, or varying degrees of visual impairment.

Differential diagnosis

The variety of the clinical syndromes that can accompany pituitary apoplexy lends itself to an array of differential diagnoses that, particularly in the absence of previous symptoms, can tax the diagnostic skill of the clinician. Thus, the precipitous escape of blood or necrotic tumour into the sub-arachnoid space can simulate an intracranial haemorrhage or an acute bacterial meningitis (Benjamin, 1929). Unilateral eye pain and an ophthalmoplegia could suggest to the unwary the presence of a berry aneurysm, whose rupture may be assumed if, in addition, there is a syndrome of meningeal irritation (Coxon, 1943; Kirschbaum and Chapman, 1948; Walton, 1953; Glass and Abbott, 1955; Walsh and Hoyt, 1969). A sudden systemic hypotension and the accompanying impaired conscious state preventing an accurate history to be taken, may simulate the myriad other causes of an unexplained low blood pressure, including myocardial disease, adrenal disturbances and, especially if accompanied by a fever, septic shock.

Pathology

Minor degenerative changes such as small cysts or areas of haemorrhage are a common microscopic feature of pituitary adenomas (Kraus, 1945). The sudden expansion of an adenoma causing pituitary apoplexy is generally thought to have a vascular cause, for the usual finding is of massive haemorrhagic necrosis of the gland with a prominence sometimes of infarction and sometimes of haemorrhage (Monro, 1913; Long, 1927; Philippides, et al, 1956; Locke and Tyler, 1961). Infarction is thought to result from tumour ischaemia due to the increased intrasellar pressure (Brougham, Heusner and Adams, 1950; List, Williams and Balyeat, 1952; Uihlein, Balfour and Donovan, 1957). Haemorrhage may result from rupture of abnormally fragile tumour vessels (Xuereb, Prichard and Daniel, 1954a; Xuereb, Prichard and Daniel, 1954b; Daniel, Prichard and Schurr, 1958). Precipitating causes have been variously cited and include radiation therapy (Bastenie, 1946; Warren, 1951; Uihlein, Balfour and Donovan, 1957; Nelson, Meakin and Dealy, 1958), hormone therapy (David, Philippon and Bernard-Weil, 1969), trauma (Reverchon, Delater and Worms, 1923; van Wagenan, 1932), hypertension (Brougham, Heusner and Adams, 1950) and anticoagulant therapy (Nourizadeh and Pitts, 1965).

Treatment (see Chapter 6)

The mortality associated with this condition is difficult to assess, for the criteria for diagnosis vary with each reported series. Furthermore, the collected cases span the pre- and post-steroid eras and, while some were treated surgically, some were not. Non-surgical management with recovery has been reported (Kreuger, Unger and Roswit, 1960) but surgical treatment is preferable for, with current microsurgical techniques, normal but compressed pituitary tissue can be identified and preserved, making replacement therapy and sterility unnecessary sequelae to the disease (Hardy et al, 1973). Sometimes even severe neurological deficits can be reversed by prompt surgical intervention (Guarnaschelli and Talalla, 1972).

CRANIOPHARYNGIOMA

Age and Sex Incidence

Craniopharyngiomas predominantly occur in the younger age groups, particularly in children. The youngest patient ever reported was a neonate in whom the tumour caused obstructive hydrocephalus (Iyer, 1952; Azar-Kia, Krishnan and Schecter, 1975). In a series of 160 patients reviewed by the author (Banna, 1973), there were three patients between two and three years of age at the time of clinical presentation. In elderly patients, the possibility of craniopharyngioma is often overlooked despite various reports emphasising that an appreciable proportion of patients show their first symptom after the age of 40 (Russell and Pennybaker, 1961). In their series of 68 patients, 24 (35 per cent) were middle-aged or elderly. In the author's series, 27 per cent were over 40 years of age and there were 14 patients (9 per cent) between 60 and 72 years at the time of presentation. In order to assess the age distribution in a larger series, about 1000 cases were collected from the literature and in these the incidence of the tumour was highest in the second decade and decreased with advancing age (Banna, 1976). Males are affected as frequently as females, but in some of the published series, there were more males than females.

Macroscopic Appearances

The majority of craniopharyngiomas arise above the sella and the rest are intrasellar in origin (Figure 5.36). An infrasellar tumour is exceedingly rare; none was found among the 160 cases reviewed by the author, but a few have been reported (Cooper and Ransohoff, 1972). About 60 per cent of craniopharyngiomas are cystic, 25 per cent are partly cystic and partly solid and only 15 per cent are completely solid. The fluid within the cyst is often yellowish-brown in colour, looking almost like fresh lubricating oil. It is rich in cholesterol crystals which give it a characteristically glittering appearance. The concentration of cholesterol within the fluid varies from case to case and may be as little as 0.07 per cent. The cyst may be unilocular or multilocular and the inner surface of its wall may be smooth or irregular. The wall of the cyst tends to adhere to the surrounding brain rendering its separation a matter of some difficulty. The solid part of the tumour may invade or infiltrate the brain and in this respect behaves like a malignant neoplasm (Figure 2.6). There is no line

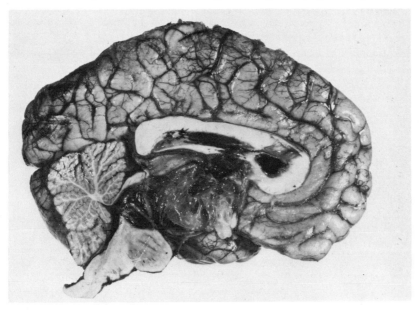

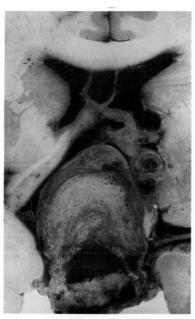

Figure 2.6. Brain invasion by craniopharyngioma. Sagittal and coronal sections of the brain of two different patients illustrating the fact that, unlike chromophobe adenoma and meningioma, there is no line of cleavage between the tumour and brain tissue. The tumour may be demarcated by reactive and adherent gliosis.

of cleavage between the tumour and the surrounding brain, but in some cases the outline of the tumour is demarcated by an area of reactive gliosis.

Microscopic Appearances

Three main types of craniopharyngioma are recognised:
1. Cystic craniopharyngioma (Figure 2.7). The cyst is lined by stratified squamous epithelium resembling the epidermis.
2. Adamantinomatous type (Figure 2.8a). The tumour is formed of fibrovascular cores

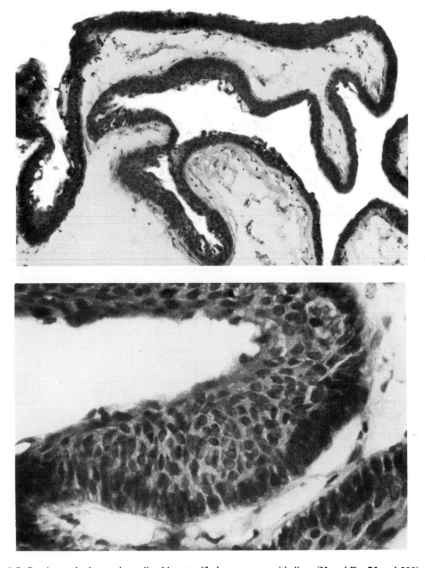

Figure 2.7. Cystic craniopharyngioma lined by stratified squamous epithelium (H and E x 75 and 500).

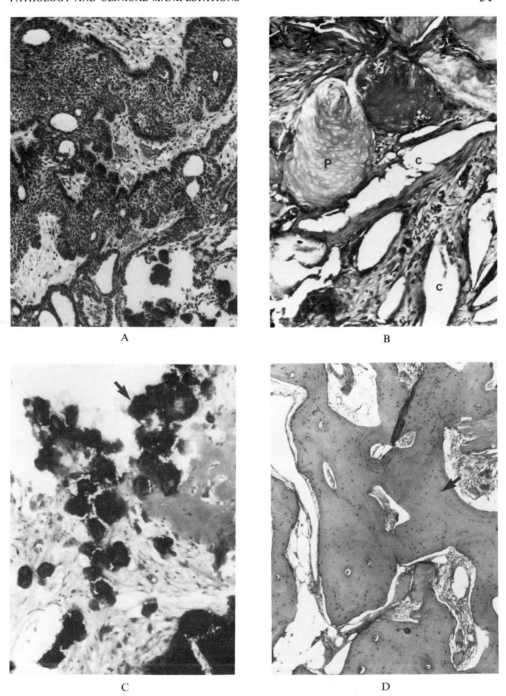

Figure 2.8. Solid craniopharyngioma. A. An epithelial core. The basal tall columnar cells resemble the amoeloblasts, hence called an adamantinomatous type of craniopharyngioma. B. Areas of coagulative necrosis. These are usually described as epithelial pearls 'p'. Numerous cholesterol clefts are present (c). C. Calcification is common (arrow). D. Bone formation is rare (arrow).

surmounted first by a layer of tall columnar cells and then by loosely packed squamous cells. The tall columnar cells resemble the adamantoblasts (ameloblasts).
3. Cysts of Rathke's cleft. This type of cyst is lined by a single layer of columnar epithelium which is often ciliated and may contain goblet cells (Figure 2.9). It is rare, accounting for approximately 4 per cent only of all craniopharyngiomas.

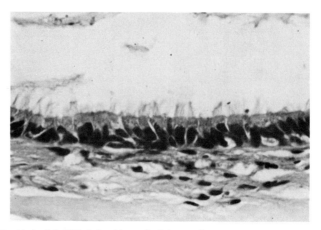

Figure 2.9. Cyst of Rathke's cleft. This is lined by a single layer of columnar ciliated epithelium.

In addition to their basic structure, various types of cellular degeneration and necrosis may occur in craniopharyngiomas. Thus, coagulative necrosis, cystic degeneration, calcification and sometimes new bone formation may be seen (Figure 2.8 b, c, d). Keratin is continuously shed from the superficial layers of the stratified squamous epithelium. In a solid tumour it appears as cholesterol clefts and in a cystic tumour, keratin gives the fluid its characteristic glittering appearance. Foreign body giant cells, lymphocytes and plasma cells may also be seen.

Craniopharyngioma is generally considered a benign neoplasm simply because the cellular structure of the tumour shows no malignant features. Nevertheless, the invasion of surrounding brain tissue by a tumour is no feature of benignity and some craniopharyngiomas ought perhaps to be considered as slowly growing locally malignant neoplasm.

Clinical Manifestations

The clinical manifestations of Rathke's pouch tumours depend to a large extent on the site of origin of the tumour, the direction of the tumour growth and its relation to the hypothalamus. (The word hypothalamus is used in its topographical sense, i.e. it includes the optic chiasm, the hypophysis cerebri, the infundibulum, the tuber cinereum, the corpora mammillaria, the posterior perforated substance as well as the hypothalamic nuclei below the hypothalamic sulcus.) Symptoms from the tumour may begin at any age, and can be divided into the following groups: (1) visual, (2) due to intracranial hypertension, (3) endocrinal, (4) personality changes, and (5) symptoms related to motor power and co-ordination.

Generally speaking, the patients' complaints vary according to their age, with a clear distinction between children and adults. In children, the first complaint is usually related to raised intracranial pressure whereas adult patients more often present with symptoms of visual impairment. Hormonal imbalance leading to disturbance in the sexual sphere is more noticeable in young adults but may be accepted by elderly patients. Personality changes are rare in the early stages of the disease but are not infrequent at a later stage, particularly in adults (patients over 16 years of age). Analysis of the clinical manifestations, based on the author's study, will now be considered in relation to the two age groups.

Clinical Manifestations of Craniopharyngiomas in Children

The clinical notes of the children at the time of their first admission to hospital were available in 67 cases. Symptoms suggestive of raised intracranial pressure (ICP) were the mode of presentation in 78 per cent of these cases. This was followed in order of frequency by visual symptoms, stunted growth, symptoms of diabetes insipidus and, rarely, weakness of one limb or one side of the body. However, on questioning and on clinical examination, manifestations of hormonal disturbances were present in 94 per cent and defective vision was discovered in 64 per cent. Attention should be drawn to the fact that frequently the presenting symptom was not the first manifestation of the disease. Retarded growth, visual defects and failure to develop secondary sexual characteristics often escape the attention of the parents who, at a later stage, are alarmed by the child's complaint of persistent headache.

Signs of raised intracranial pressure

Children who sought medical advice because of headache constituted approximately 66 per cent of the cases. Headache is often intermittent. The child wakes up with pain in the head, which is described as throbbing or a dull ache, lasts for a few hours and gradually passes away. The duration of the attack varies and may be as little as 10 to 15 minutes. It may be repeated every day or may be in the early stages of the disease, occurring about once or twice a month. This situation may persist without causing undue concern for periods extending to a number of years. The onset of an attack is usually paroxysmal, but as it passes away it often leaves a mild residual pain. Between attacks, the child may be perfectly normal.

Vomiting in association with headache occurred in about 30 per cent of the cases, but in another 4 per cent vomiting was the main complaint. It may be severe and projectile, occurring more frequently on rising in the morning, but in many cases the child is only said to be 'off his food'. Examination of the optic fundi is usually difficult in children. Nevertheless, papilloedema was detected in 31 per cent of the cases and of these 4 per cent had no symptoms of raised ICP.

Endocrinal abnormalities

Stunted growth was obvious to the parents in about 7 per cent of the cases, but retarded bone age of varying severity on x-ray examination was present in 41 per cent. In three children aged 8, 11 and 12 years there was 50 per cent retardation of skeletal maturation. Precocity is rare with craniopharyngiomas, but occurred in three male children aged 3, 4 and 7 years, the 7-year-old boy showing sexual characteristics. Obesity was an outstanding feature in six children (9 per cent); five males and one female. Another six children were described as small, thin and fragile, of the 'Lorain type' of panhypopituitarism. Poor sexual development occurred in about 20 per cent of the children who were about the age of puberty at the time of presentation, but in female children a delayed menarche was always present. Symptoms of diabetes insipidus in the form of excessive thirst or polyuria were the initial complaints of five children (7 per cent) and these manifestations were noted in one other child on admission.

Visual disturbances

Visual defects were found on clinical examination in 43 children (64 per cent), of whom one-third complained of visual difficulties. Of four children with diplopia, three had papilloedema and abducens palsy, and the fourth had a convergent squint but no papilloedema. Horizontal nystagmus was detected in two children and a third child had see-saw nystagmus. All three showed evidence of raised ICP.

Muscle power and co-ordination

Monoplegia or hemiplegia was present in four children and unsteadiness of gait was noted in seven. In one, the ataxia was thought to be due to defective vision.

Psychological disorders and level of consciousness

Two children were described as abnormally quiet and of slow mentality. A third was said to be an aggressive pituitary dwarf and a fourth child was transferred initially from the school psychological service on account of her extreme shyness and withdrawn behaviour. She was subsequently found to have an abnormal skull radiograph. Repeated loss of consciousness occurred in one patient and four others were admitted in a state of collapse. Six children were described as somnolent.

Clinical Manifestations of Craniopharyngiomas in Adults

Visual failure was the main presenting symptom in about 80 per cent of the cases. This was followed in order of frequency by headache, personality change, symptoms of diabetes insipidus and gonadal dysfunction. About 5 per cent of the patients were stuporose or unconscious on admission.

Visual disturbances

Many patients first presented themselves to the optician or the ophthalmologist, having noticed that their visual acuity was deteriorating. Other visual symptoms pointed directly to a lesion compressing the optic chiasm. Examples of such symptoms were not infrequent. The patient might state that he had difficulty in seeing properly to either side, as if he were wearing blinkers. Others complained that in reading they could not find the end or the beginning of the line clearly — the words at both ends appeared wiped off. Among other visual complaints the following are quoted in the patients' own words:
'I cannot read because the lines are jumbled together, they are fused and irregular.'
'I cannot see red very clearly and have trouble in seeing the traffic lights.'
'Part of my eye is opaque', or 'There is a smoke screen or black lace in front of my eyes.'
One patient complained of occasional purple spots in front of his eyes. A few patients had double vision; as in the patient who said, 'I see double when I look ahead, with the images

side by side. Sometimes the two images overlap, as when I saw two buses which later fused.' Double vision was transient and fluctuating in one case.

On examination, visual abnormalities were present in 76 patients, i.e. 93 per cent of the cases. In these, varying degrees of optic atrophy were noted in 35 (46 per cent) and papilloedema in 9 patients only (12 per cent). Examination of the visual fields showed bitemporal field defects in 23 patients (30 per cent). This was usually in the form of an incomplete hemianopia with scattered areas of scotoma in the remaining part of the field. In early cases where the defect was limited to one quadrant, no significant preponderance of upper or lower quadrantanopia could be established. At the time of presentation more than one quadrant of the field was usually involved. Concentric diminution in the visual field was reported in three patients (4 per cent), of whom one was left with central vision only. Homonymous hemianopia occurred in five patients (7 per cent) indicating that the tumour had involved the optic tract. Blindness of one eye or severe deterioration of vision in both eyes amounting to blindness was noted in seven patients (9 per cent). It is important to draw attention to the fact that some patients with blindness in one eye may remain unaware of their disability until vision in the other eye begins to deteriorate. Central or centro-caecal scotoma without involvement of the peripheral field occurred in seven cases (9 per cent). This type of visual abnormality was often thought to be due to a variety of conditions including retrobulbar neuritis, vitamin B_{12} deficiency or tobacco amblyopia. Squint was rare and occurred in three patients, of whom none had papilloedema, being a convergent squint in one case. A fourth patient had unilateral ptosis and a fifth complained of severe peri-orbital pain in one eye, which was later shown to be due to extension of the tumour. Of all the 82 patients in the series, only six had no abnormality on fundal or visual field examination.

The duration of symptoms before seeking medical advice was available in 60 patients. It was less than one year in 45 patients (75 per cent), between 2 and 5 years in ten (17 per cent), about 7 years in one and in two patients over 70 years of age, visual impairment was present for many years before admission. Sudden loss of vision, suggestive of vascular disease, was reported in two patients.

Mental symptoms

Mental deterioration in association with craniopharyngioma occurred in 22 patients (26 per cent), in ten of whom it occurred prior to any other symptom. Among the remaining 12 patients, one became mentally disabled 14 years following irradiation treatment and a second became vague, sleepy and apathetic following surgery. Symptoms of mental deterioration in the present series can be roughly divided into four types:

Dementia. Severe mental deterioration with disorientation in time and space was evident in seven patients, i.e. about 8 per cent of the cases. In addition to being confused, some patients were extremely sleepy during the day and noisy during the night. Some were so demented that they did not know their age, their year or their country of origin. Writing alphabetical letters was impossible in a number of cases. All the patients in this group showed varying degrees of ventricular dilatation. This dilatation in some cases was secondary to a small tumour obstructing the foramen of Monro, but large tumours infiltrating the corpus callosum and the frontal lobes were more liable to produce symptoms of mental deterioration.

Amnesia. Loss of memory for recent events was an important symptom of craniopharyngioma in six patients (7 per cent). This was often associated with a mild to moderate degree of intellectual impairment. Recent or short-term memory was invariably affected, but remote or long-term memory was often less involved. In one patient, signs of an organic Korsakow's psychosis were described. In this group of patients, the tumour growth was mostly in a posterior direction, towards the brain stem and the hippocampus. The aqueduct was often displaced posteriorly, but was not necessarily obstructed. Ventricular dilatation occurred in three out of six patients.

Depression. A clinical picture simulating depression was noted in six patients (7 per cent). These patients complained of being excessively tired and sleepy. They became disinterested and lost concentration. On examination, they were found to be dull, lethargic and apathetic. One patient was described as being irritable and confused in addition to being depressed. Four patients in this group showed evidence of ventricular dilatation.

Minor intellectual impairment. Mild intellectual deterioration occurred in three patients (3.5 per cent). In all of them the cerebral ventricles were enlarged.

Hormonal disturbances

The earliest and most common hormonal disturbances were related to the gonadotrophic hormones. Of the female patients, 60% within the fertility age admitted to having menstrual irregularities for many years prior to the development of visual symptoms. In male patients, loss of libido was present in about 30 per cent, but few of them admitted to impotence. Adiposity was the second most frequent manifestation. About 17 per cent of the patients were said to be obese. Diabetes insipidus was present in 13 patients (16 per cent), but only eight complained initially of this symptom. The remaining five patients admitted to polydipsia and polyuria on questioning. Panhypopituitarism occurred in six patients (7 per cent). One patient was treated for hypothyroidism for six years before she was admitted as an emergency in an unconscious state and was found to have a craniopharyngioma.

Headache and raised intracranial pressure

Headache was present in about 36 patients (44 per cent), but papilloedema was discovered in only 12 (15 per cent) and sellar changes of raised ICP in 8 (10 per cent). Headache was often due to the presence of the tumour and was not necessarily indicative of ventricular dilatation.

Symptoms related to muscular power and co-ordination

Unsteadiness of gait was present in two patients. In the second, ataxia was associated with unilateral disturbance of the eighth nerve by extension of the tumour into the cerebello-pontine angle. Pyramidal signs were present in four patients, of whom three showed weakness and spasticity of the lower limbs and one had a hemiparesis. In a fifth case the tumour occurred in a patient suffering from peroneal muscular atrophy.

SUPRASELLAR MENINGIOMA

The term meningioma was introduced by Cushing (1922) to describe a benign intracranial neoplasm which for centuries had been given different and often confusing names including epithelioma, sarcoma, fibroblastoma, mesothelioma, endothelioma and psammoma. The word meningioma itself is non-committal and simply indicates that the tumour arises from the meninges. However, its use has persisted and it is now generally accepted that meningiomas are of arachnoid cell origin and probably arise from the arachnoid granulations or villi, which are most common in relation to the superior sagittal sinus, the commonest site of origin of meningiomas. The distribution of arachnoid granulations at the base of the brain is shown in Figure 2.10. They are most numerous in relation to the cavernous and the sphenoparietal venous sinuses, hence the preponderance of sphenoidal ridge meningiomas among meningiomas of the skull base. The arachnoid granulations were first described by Antonio Pacchioni in 1697 (Garrison, 1929). They are very small in children, but can be identified on close inspection from about the age of 18 months and at the age of three years they are disseminated over a considerable area and increase in number and size with advancing age.

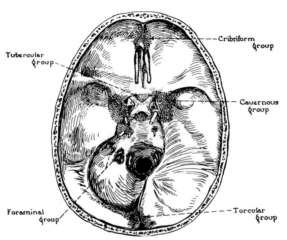

Figure 2.10. Location of arachnoid granulations over base of skull. Note they are abundant in the parasellar region in relation to the cavernous and spheno-parietal sinuses. (After Aoyagi, T. and Kyuno, K., Tokyo, 1912.)

Age and Sex Incidence

Meningiomas are tumours of adult life and are seldom seen in children. They reach a peak incidence in patients 40 to 50 years of age, and are more common in females, although the sex incidence varies in tumours at different sites. In the sellar region, they are three to four times more common in women. Meningiomas constitute approximately 15 per cent of all intracranial neoplasms, but the sellar region is one of the less common sites. It gives rise to approximately 2.3 per cent (Traub, 1961) to 7 per cent (Banna and Appleby, 1969) of all intracranial meningiomas.

Macroscopic Appearance

Meningiomas are encapsulated tumours which invaginate, but do not invade the brain. They are usually attached to the dura mater and receive part of their blood supply from the meningeal arteries and part from contiguous cerebral vessels. They are usually firm in con-

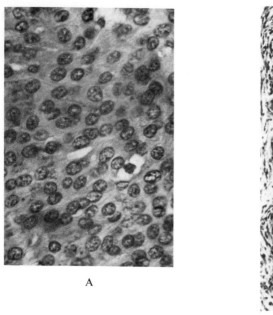

A

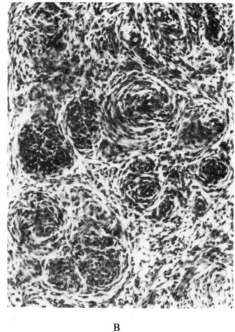

B

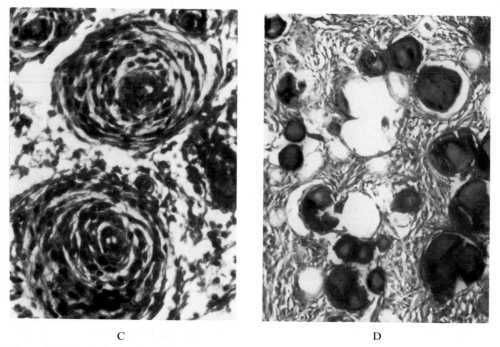

C   D

Figure 2.11. Classical microscopic appearances of meningioma. A, Meningothelial or syncytial. B and C, Transitional. D, Psammomatous. E, Fibroblastic. F, Angioblastic.

sistency, have a finely granular cut surface and can be separated easily from the surrounding brain. Occasionally, they are soft and separation is more difficult. Localised thickening of the skull bones, when present, is an important feature of meningioma. It may occur as a result of penetration of the dura mater by the tumour and by invasion of the overlying bone, with ossification of the stroma of the invading tumour, but it may be found in the absence of bone infiltration and is then believed to be due to increased vascularity leading to osteoblastic activity. New bone formation may be extensive in meningiomas spreading over the surface of the brain as in meningioma en plaque and sometimes it may be responsible for most of the patient's symptoms, particularly if it encroaches upon the foramina at the base of the skull. In a few cases meningiomas may be associated with pressure erosion or destruction of the overlying bone.

Microscopic Appearances

There are various classifications of meningiomas and as many as nine types and 20 subtypes have been described (Cushing and Eisenhardt, 1938), but the main groups are (Figure 2.11):

1. Meningothelial or syncytial meningioma. In this type, the tumour is formed of solid masses or sheets of polygonal cells with ill-defined cell outlines and regular oval nuclei.
2. Transitional meningioma. Here the cells are arranged concentrically and are wrapped around each other forming whorls. The tendency for whorl formation varies from one tumour to another and in different parts of the same tumour. Hyaline degeneration and calcification of the whorls give rise to the psammoma bodies (psammos = sand). When these are abundant the tumour is described as a psammomatous meningioma.

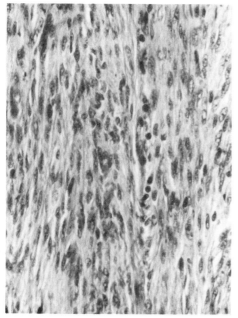

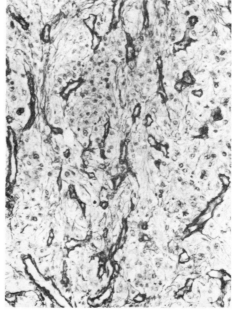

E   F

3. Fibroblastic meningioma. In this type the tumour is formed of interlacing bundles of long spindle cells with abundant collagen and reticular fibres.
4. Angiomatous meningioma. As the name implies the tumour is very vascular and contains numerous thin-walled vessels. It tends to be more aggressive and recurs more frequently than the average meningioma (Rubinstein, 1972).

Of the four main groups, the first and second are the commonest, but mixed types are frequently seen. Other rare varieties include melanotic, sarcomatous, lipomatous, osteoblastic and chondroblastic meningiomas.

Clinical Manifestations

Meningiomas in the sellar area are often relatively small and they seldom, if ever, acquire the size of a 'massive' chromophobe adenoma or craniopharyngioma. Nevertheless, they have a notorious tendency to wrap themselves around nerves and blood vessels at the base of the brain, rendering complete surgical removal impractical. The majority of patients present with visual failure, and in them optic atrophy is common. Paralysis of the ocular muscles may occur if the superior orbital fissure is narrowed by a new bone formation or, less frequently, by tumour extension into the orbit. Vascular occlusions may lead to cortical motor and sensory manifestations, but because the occlusion occurs very gradually over many months or years, it may be totally asymptomatic and come to light only at angiography. Meningiomas are said to increase in size during menstruation or pregnancy, hence the patient's symptoms may fluctuate during the course of the disease (Bickerstaff, Small and Guest, 1958). Endocrine dysfunction, if present, is usually less apparent than in pituitary adenoma or craniopharyngioma.

OPTIC NERVE GLIOMA

Age and Sex Incidence

Gliomas of the optic nerve and chiasm (Figure 2.12) are rare tumours that constitute approximately 3.5 per cent of all intracranial tumours in children, less than 1 per cent of intracranial tumours in adults and about 2 per cent of orbital tumours in all age groups. Very few of these tumours are confined to one optic nerve. The chiasm and one or both optic nerves and adjacent brain are usually involved from the time of initial diagnosis (Reese, 1963). There is a disproportionately high incidence of optic nerve glioma in childhood so much so that a congenital origin of these tumours has been suggested. About 80 per cent occur in children less than 10 years of age (Schuster and Westberg, 1967) and there are many reports in the literature (Marshall, 1954) which indicate a common association of these tumours with multiple neurofibromatosis (von Recklinghausen's disease). The incidence of café-au-lait spots, with or without other neurological manifestations, is quoted by various authors as 17 per cent, 37.5 per cent and 100 per cent (Ladekarl, 1964).

Microscopic Appearances

Histologically (Figure 2.12B) the majority of these tumours are astrocytomas grade I or II. A few are probably oligodendrogliomas, but grade III and IV astrocytomas rarely affect the optic nerve and if they do, it is usually in an adult (Henderson, 1973). Some tumours are described as spongioblastoma or piloid astrocytoma but, regardless of the nomenclature,

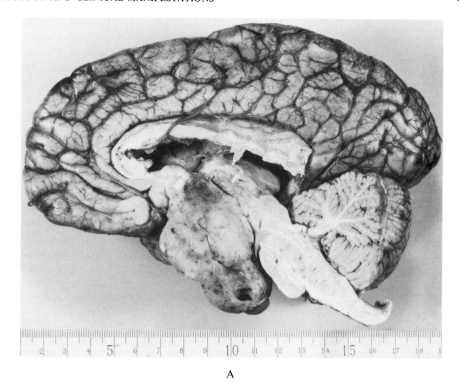

A

Figure 2.12 A. Juvenile astrocytoma of the hypothalamus. This midsagittal section of the tumour demonstrates a large mass anterior to the pons. It is well circumscribed in most places except for infiltration of the hypothalamus. It is mostly solid, focally haemorrhagic and cystic in its most dependent portion. B. Histological section of an optic chiasm glioma with residual pattern of the optic nerve. (By courtesy of Dr L. J. Rubinstein.)

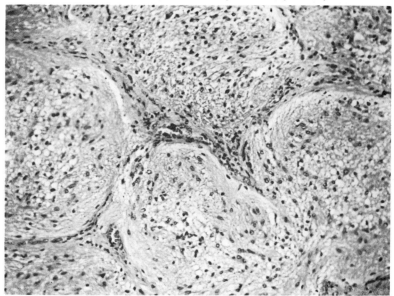

B

there are two important facts on which most pathologists seem to agree. First, the majority of optic nerve gliomas occurring in children are of low grade malignancy, whereas in adults they are more aggressive and malignant (Hoyt et al, 1973). Secondly, the further the tumour extends centripetally towards the optic chiasm, the less histologically benign it is said to be (Slooff and Slooff, 1975).

Clinical Manifestations

The clinical manifestations of optic nerve glioma depend on whether the tumour arises within or behind the orbit. In general, the intraorbital lesions present with proptosis, ipsilateral loss of vision, strabismus and papilloedema, in that order of frequency (Dodge et al, 1958). The intradural lesions lead to loss of vision in both eyes in more than 90 per cent of cases and may be associated with symptoms of obstructive hydrocephalus or hypothalamic dysfunction. In young patients, slight visual impairment may not be noted by the parents. Among 36 cases reported by Hoyt and Baghdassarian (1969) there were nine children in whom the tumour was identified in the course of paediatric and radiological investigations for non-ocular problems such as plexiform facial neuroma, ataxia, mental retardation, diabetes insipidus, hydrocephalus, neonatal jaundice and precocious puberty. The latter was present in eight patients in whom seven had neurofibromatosis. Amongst the cases, one glioma was found incidentally in a 64-year-old woman, but this must be extremely rare.

HYPOTHALAMIC GLIOMA

Hypothalamic glioma occurs primarily in young patients, hence it is often known as juvenile astrocytoma of the hypothalamus (Rubinstein, 1972). The tumour arises in the floor or the walls of the third ventricle and may infiltrate downwards into the optic chiasm or upwards into the thalamus and towards the interventricular foramen. It is a slowly growing tumour which may appear circumscribed to the naked eye and may be cystic or solid; the cysts may be large or small. During the present study, the case of a young man 32 years of age was studied. His skull radiographs showed an abnormal pituitary fossa and suprasellar curvilinear calcification which was thought radiologically and on exploration to be a craniopharyngioma. On aspirating the cyst, however, there was no glitter of cholesterol crystals, but a protein rich coagulating fluid of a malignant tumour. Biopsy of the cyst wall confirmed the diagnosis of cystic astrocytoma.

Clinical Manifestations

Juvenile astrocytoma of the hypothalamus may cause hypothalamic dysfunction in the early stages of the disease, which may not be severe enough to lead the patient to seek medical advice. One of our patients weighed about 130 kg and was known to have had an excessive appetite for many years. It was because of symptoms resulting from ventricular obstruction however, that he saw his family doctor. Patients with this type of lesion may, on the other hand, suffer from extreme emaciation and diabetes insipidus and may present with visual failure. In infants, hypothalamic glioma should also be considered as one of the possible causes of the diencephalic syndrome (Girwood and Ross, 1969; Addy and Hudson, 1972; Danziger and Bloch, 1974).

CHORDOMA

Chordomas are relatively rare tumours, probably arising from remnants of the notochord, the forerunner of the axial skeleton. Despite their embryonic origin, only a few cases have been reported in children (Becker et al, 1975). The majority occur in patients 30 to 50 years of age. Another strange feature of these tumours is that they are very rare in the dorsal and lumbar parts of the vertebral column which contain the largest portion of the nucleus pulposus, the remains of the notochord. Approximately 50 per cent of chordomas arise in the sacro-coccygeal region, 35 per cent are found in the base of the skull and the remaining 15 per cent occur in the cervical, lumbar and thoracic spine, in that order of frequency (Dahlin and MacCarty, 1952). Most intracranial chordomas occur in the mid-line in the region of the basisphenoid. They usually grow forward along the base of the skull but growth in other directions is known to occur. One probably unique case of intrasellar chordoma has been reported (Mathews and Wilson, 1974). In this case the tumour probably arose from a purely intrasellar ectopic vestigium of the notochord.

From an historical point of view and according to Adson, Kernohan and Woltman (1935): 'This tumour was first reported by Luschka who in 1856 described small mucus-containing excrescences which protruded from the basisphenoid and perforated the dura mater. The next year, Virchow saw similar nodules and designated them "ecchordosis physaliphora" (derived from the Greek words: ek = out, chordo = cord, osis = a disease process and physallis = bubble). In 1838 Müller suggested that these masses originated from remnants of the notochord which they resembled histologically, and also traced the notochord up to the sella turcica. Similar masses were frequently seen during the next 35 years, and in 1894 Ribbert and Steiner found five examples of these masses. In 1895 Ribbert proved that they were of notochord origin and suggested that tumours originated from them should be called chordomas. Most of the early examples of chordomas were found at necropsy and had not given rise to clinical symptoms.'

Macroscopic Appearance

The tumour is soft, lobulated and jelly-like in consistency. It may be colourless or greyish-white depending on its cellularity and mucin content. Areas of haemorrhage and calcification may be present. The tumour is usually well demarcated yet invasive and cannot be totally removed. Intracranially, it usually arises from the clivus and is mid-line in position, but it may extend entirely to one side. It may grow upwards towards the sella, forwards into the nasopharynx or backwards towards the brain stem producing a wide variety of clinical signs. Metastases from intracranial chordomas practically never occur, although there are a few reports of metastases from chordomas in the sacro-coccygeal region.

Microscopic Appearance

Lobulation and a cord-like arrangement of tumour cells are usually evident on microscopic examination. The most characteristic feature is the presence of mucin inside the tumour cells, in the extracellular space or within the cell nuclei. During histological preparation mucin dissolves, appearing as vacuoles and giving rise to the characteristic physaliform cells of a chordoma (Figure 2.13).

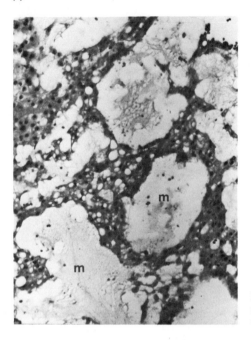

Figure 2.13. Chordoma. Note excessive mucinous material within the cells (physaliform cells) and in the extracellular spaces.

Clinical Manifestations

The most common symptoms of clivus chordoma are headache, visual disturbances, nasal obstruction (from ventral extension of the tumour into the nasopharynx) and pain in the neck (Givner, 1945). Diplopia due to paralysis of the lateral rectus muscle, less frequently of the medial rectus, occurs in about one-third of the cases. Visual field defects, optic atrophy or papilloedema due to compression of the optic chiasm are also common. Although the tumour is typically a mid-line lesion, there is a pronounced tendency for involvement of the cranial nerves to be unilateral and even if the involvement is bilateral, it is more complete or widespread on one side than the other. The visual field defects are similar to those caused by other lesions in the sellar region, but in chordoma, functional disturbance of the hypophysis is rare and occurs later in the course of the disease. Headache usually precedes changes in the visual fields which is the reversal of its sequence in pituitary tumours.

In addition to the abducent, the trochlear, the oculomotor and the optic nerves, practically any cranial nerve may be involved. Chordoma may present as a cerebello-pontine angle tumour affecting primarily the acoustic, the vestibular and the facial nerves. It may present as a lesion in the region of the jugular fossa involving the glossopharyngeal, vagus and accessory nerves and further extension may involve the hypoglossal canal and the foramen magnum, the latter resulting in neck stiffness and pain accentuated by head movement. Second in frequency to cranial nerve palsies are the symptoms and signs resulting from compression and displacement of the pons, medulla or upper part of the cervical cord. They include long tract sensory and motor disturbances in addition to involvement of cranial nerve nuclei.

ANEURYSM

The association between aneurysms and tumours in the sellar region may be encountered in three situations:

1. As an incidental lesion coexisting with any pituitary lesion. One such case was reported by Lippman, Onofrio and Baker (1971). We also have had two cases and know of others unpublished.
2. Aneurysms presenting as a tumour compressing the optic nerve or chiasm (see radiology section).
3. As a cause of hypopituitarism – a very rare presentation of an aneurysm. White and Ballantine (1961) were able to collect 35 cases from the literature and since then a few others have been added (Cartlidge and Shaw, 1972). Amenorrhoea, impotence, diabetes insipidus, somnolence, panhypopituitarism and severe adrenocortical insufficiency were all reported in patients with aneurysms. Severe adrenocortical insufficiency leading to coma and successfully treated with steroids, may develop suddenly upon rupture of the aneurysm (Cartlidge and Shaw, 1972).

Aneurysms causing direct compression of the pituitary gland arise from the infraclinoid part of the internal carotid artery and point towards the sella, which may be normal or enlarged in a fashion often described previously as 'classical' of pituitary adenoma. In fact, one of the cases illustrated by White and Ballantine (1961) showed a sella which expanded on sequential radiographs similar to an enlarging pituitary adenoma. Visual symptoms may be absent in these cases. On the other hand, aneurysms arising from the anterior part of the circle of Willis, or rarely from the tip of the basilar artery and indirectly compressing the gland from above, are invariably associated with visual field defects. It would be reassuring to think that aneurysms can be ruled out by angiography, but unfortunately, this is not true. There are exceptionally rare cases where an aneurysm, totally occupied by organised thrombus, fails to opacify on angiography. White and Ballantine (1961) concluded that some of the clinical manifestations which may help to warn the surgeon that an expanding intrasellar mass is probably an aneurysm rather than a pituitary tumour are:

1. Abrupt onset of symptoms.
2. Sudden severe headache, suggestive of leakage of blood.
3. Supra-orbital pain.
4. Neurological evidence of compression of the third, fourth, fifth and sixth cranial nerves.
5. Monocular blindness, especially when there is no cut in the temporal field of the opposite eye.
6. Bizarre changes in the visual fields, especially a nasal defect in the eye on the side of the aneurysm, with or without a cut in the opposite temporal field, or an inferior altitudinal hemianopsia.

CHOLESTEATOMA (dermoid and epidermoid cysts)

Cholesteatomas, not due to infective middle-ear diseases, are rare intracranial tumours probably developmental in origin. They were first reported by Cruveilhier, who in 1829 described a growth found at the base of the brain displacing the third ventricle superiorly and extending as far anteriorly as the sella turcica. Because of the external glistening silvery appearance of the tumour, he called it a 'pearly tumour'. Müller (1838) reported two examples and because their contents had all the features of cholesterin he called them cholesteatoma. Virchow (1855) discussed a number of these cases but, because he failed to demonstrate cholesterin in all of them, believed the term 'pearly tumour' to be more suitable. The origin of these tumours remained obscure until 1854, when von Remak suggested that they might arise from misplaced epithelial tissue. This work was substantiated by Bostroem who in 1897 introduced the term 'pial epidermoid' to indicate their origin from embryonic skin elements at a comparatively late stage, whereas the pial dermoids arise from cell rests included earlier in embryonic life (Tytus and Pennybacker, 1956).

The main tumour mass is made up of epithelial debris which slowly accumulates within the capsule from desquamating cells of the epithelial lining. It contains fatty caseous material and cholesterol and its consistency depends upon the proportion of these substances. The capsule of an epidermoid consists of an epidermal layer without dermal structures (Figure 2.14) whereas a dermoid capsule is composed of epidermis, together with a dermal layer containing hair and sebaceous glands. Both types are similar to the naked eye, and since their

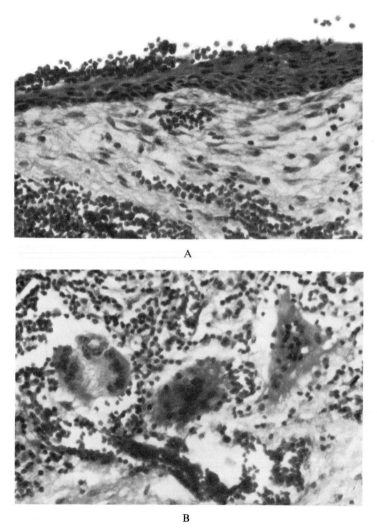

A

B

Figure 2.14. Cholesteatoma. A. In the above case the tumour capsule is formed of a thin layer of keratinizing squamous cells. B. Multiple giant cells are present in many parts of the tumour capsule.

characteristics are the same as regards growth, recurrence and complications, many authors consider a sharp distinction between the two to be unnecessary (Tytus and Pennybacker, 1956). They are both non-neoplastic, encapsulated and very slow growing. They do not invade the surrounding brain, but infiltration and malignancy have been reported in a few cases in the literature. These were probably terato-dermoids rather than dermoids; differentiation between the two lesions may occasionally be difficult.

Intracranially, these tumours commonly occur in the posterior fossa particularly in the cerebello-pontine angle. However, they have been reported in other sites including the middle cranial fossa, the sellar region and within the lateral ventricles (Banna, 1976). Clinically, there are no features which distinguish cholesteatoma from other tumours in the sellar area. In a recent case, the tumour was an incidental finding in a patient who was being investigated for dementia (Figure 5.10d).

SUPRASELLAR GERMINOMA (dysgerminoma, ectopic pinealoma, teratoid or atypical teratoma)

Dysgerminoma is a rare but well recognised malignant ovarian tumour, histologically very similar in appearance to the seminoma; it is thought to arise from residual, potentially 'male' germ cells in the ovary. The main characteristic features of these tumours are their homogeneous pinkish colour and uniform cellular structure of rounded polygonal cells with central nuclei and variable lymphocytic infiltration around a fibrous stroma which divides the tumour into irregular lobules. Very occasionally tumours of similar microscopic structure are found intracranially, usually in the region of the pineal body and rarely in relation to the hypothalamus. They occur predominantly in males, 10 to 30 years of age and reach a peak incidence in the latter half of the second decade. Those occurring in the suprasellar region have been classified, with regard to their location and clinical presentation, into three types (Kageyama and Belsky, 1961).

The first type occurs together with a similar tumour in the pineal body, but either one or the other may appear first. Whether the sellar lesion is a seeding metastasis or due to multifocality is not known. The patient may present with visual manifestations of a pineal body tumour (Parinaud's syndrome), chiasmal compression, hydrocephalus or hypo-pituitarism and may be occasionally difficult to differentiate from glioma of the optic chiasm (Cohen, Steinberg and Buchwald, 1974).

The second type is the ectopic pinealoma which arises in the third ventricle, primarily involving the hypothalamus and leading to ventricular obstruction. Diabetes insipidus is an initial symptom and may be the only symptom for many years. Visual failure and hypopituitarism develop at a later stage.

The third type is an ectopic pinealoma located mainly beneath the cerebral hemispheres in the region of the optic chiasm which may extend into the pituitary fossa. In these cases manifestations of chiasmal compression and hypopituitarism occur early and ventricular dilatation is absent. There are some cases reported of intrasellar germinomas arising primarily within the sella in which the presenting symptoms are related to hypofunction of the pituitary gland (Ghatak, Hirano and Zimmerman, 1969).

As stated earlier, this tumour has a distinctive histological appearance, being composed of two types of cells (Rubinstein, 1972): large polygonal cells with well defined cell membrane, pale eosinophilic cytoplasm and conspicuous central nuclei; and groups of small darkly staining cells, presumably lymphocytes, usually distributed along the vascular connective tissue stroma of the tumour (Figure 2.15). A true teratoma containing many kinds of tissue of endodermal, mesodermal and ectodermal origin is extremely rare in the sellar area, but is known to occur in the pineal region. With occasional exceptions, pineal teratomas affect

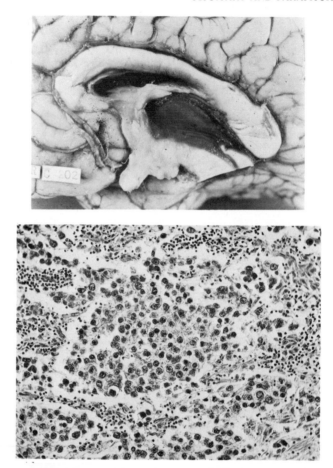

Figure 2.15. Suprasellar germinoma. Gross photograph: This 19-year-old man had a 4-year history of diabetes insipidus, followed one year later by panhypopituitarism. At post mortem, the optic chiasm, pituitary stalk and hypothalamus were diffusely infiltrated by an ill-defined, firm, greyish tumour. The presence of fresh blood in the lateral ventricle and in the dilated third ventricle is due to recent surgical trauma. Photomicrograph: Microscopic appearances of tumour infiltrating the hypothalamus, illustrated in the previous gross photograph. The tumour consists of two distinct cell types: large spheroidal cells with central vesiculated nuclei resembling those of the testicular seminoma and ovarian dysgerminoma, and lymphocytes. No transitional forms are seen between the two cell types. Haematoxylin and eosin x 130. (Reproduced from Rubinstein, 1972 with kind permission.)

males and in about half of the cases are accompanied by precocious bodily and sexual development (Willis, 1962).

HYPOTHALAMIC HAMARTOMA

This is a developmental tumour occurring in the posterior part of the hypothalamus, behind the dorsum sellae and closely related to the floor of the third ventricle. Few cases have been reported, of which the majority were in male children and the main presenting feature was precocious puberty both in physical and sexual development, associated with mental retardation in one of the cases reported (Northfield and Russell, 1967), but in another case the tumour was discovered as a chance finding in a previously normal individual (Wolman and Balmforth, 1963). The tumour is usually small in size, about 1.0 to 2.0 cm in diameter, and is situated in the cisterna interpeduncularis. Because of its location in the basal cisterns, it can be readily demonstrated by pneumoencephalography (Figure 2.16). Skull radiographs and carotid angiograms may be normal in these cases and ventriculography may fail to demonstrate the lesion or it may show a filling defect in the floor of the third ventricle which is indistinguishable from that due to a malignant tumour in that region. To the naked eye the tumour is encapsulated and firm and has a coarsely lobulated, smooth glistening surface. It may be adherent to the tuber cinereum and to the mammillary bodies. Histologically, it is composed of a haphazard assembly of neurones, bundles of nerve fibres and neurological cells (Figure 2.17), but mature nerve cells of different size and shape may be present (Northfield and Russell, 1967).

INFUNDIBULOMA

Infundibuloma is an uncommon tumour arising primarily from the neurohypophysis. Both clinically and radiologically it is indistinguishable from other tumours occurring in the hypothalamic area in childhood. Pathologically on the other hand, it has a fairly characteristic appearance (Wolman, 1959). The tumour is large, fleshy, nodular and has a bluish tinge. The cut surface shows a variegated pink and yellow appearance with cyst formation of varying size. Histologically (Figure 2.18), the tumour is characterised by:
1. A vascular pattern in the form of aggregations of thin-walled vessels, many of which appear to branch or coil in a corkscrew manner which has a striking resemblance to the hypophyseal portal system. In addition, there are many vascular, sinusoidal channels filled with blood or serous fluid.
2. The tumour is composed of fusiform cells with unipolar or bipolar processes that resemble the pituicytes.
3. The presence of multiple eosinophilic colloidal bodies or droplets which are probably degenerative glial fibres.

MYOBLASTOMA

The granular cell myoblastoma is a benign tumour occurring within the striated muscle of the tongue but it has also been reported in the subcutaneous tissue, the gastrointestinal tract, omentum, retroperitoneum, bladder, larynx and breast. It may occur very rarely in the region of the pituitary gland, infundibulum and hypothalamus. According to Kobrine and Ross (1973), only 12 cases have so far been described in the literature; the first was in 1893 by Boyce and Beadles and the second 28 years later. Kobrine and Ross (1973) reviewed all 12 cases and discussed the possible aetiology of the tumour. Microscopically the lesion consists of large, regular polygonal cells with faintly granular, eosinophilic cytoplasm. In the pituitary region the tumour probably arises from ectopic 'myoblastomatous' cells. Aggregates of these cells may be found in about 10 per cent of normal pituitary glands (Doron, Behar and Beller, 1965) and small tumours may be discovered incidentally at postmortem examination (Rubinstein, 1972). Some authors considered the tumour a hamartoma and named it 'choristoma', meaning a mass of tissue histologically normal for an organ or part of the body other than the site at which it is located. Others thought the tumour

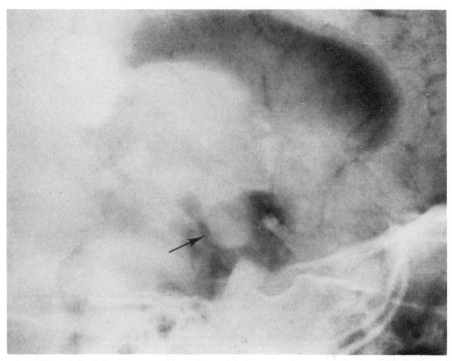

Figure 2.16. Hypothalamic hamartoma. This radiograph belongs to a four-year-old male child who had a bone age of 12 years and showed marked precocious sexual tendencies and secondary sexual characteristics. He had a high plasma level of androgenic steroids, all other tests were normal. The tumour is outlined by air in the interpeduncular cistern at pneumoencephalography. (By courtesy of Dr David J. Zacks.)

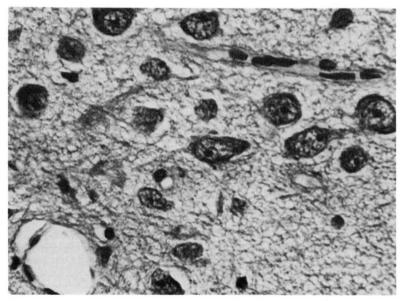

Figure 2.17. Photomicrograph of a hypothalamic hamartoma: The tissue contains mature nerve cells, varying considerably in size and shape and dispersed fairly evenly throughout all areas (H and E x 500). (By courtesy of Mr D. W. C. Northfield and the editor of *Journal of Neurology, Neurosurgery and Psychiatry.*)

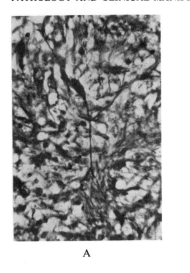

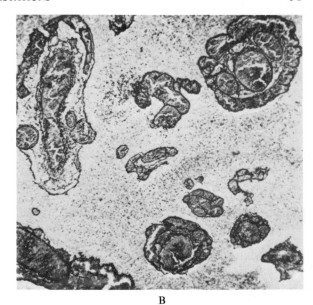

Figure 2.18. Infundibuloma. A. Unipolar cell with elongated slender process which bifurcates. Silver carbonate (x 250). B. Glomerular-like collections of vessels in tumour. Reticulin and Masson trichrome (x 60). (By kind permission of the editor of the *Journal of Pathology and Bacteriology*.)

to be of neuroglial origin and that it should be termed 'pituicytoma', while a third and more recent view is in favour of a Schwann cell origin.

Of the 12 cases reported in the literature (Kobrine and Ross, 1973), there were eight females and four males, ranging in age from 27 to 69 years. The commonest presenting complaint was deterioration of vision. Three patients presented with headache only and one with memory loss. Endocrine disturbances were present in eight patients and the duration of symptoms ranged from two weeks to five years. The skull radiographs showed non-specific sellar changes in eight and absence of calcification in all the cases. The findings on air study were similar to those found in other suprasellar tumours, but 'tumour stain' was demonstrated at angiography in four out of six cases; a feature, as we shall see later in the radiology section; primarily of meningioma, it is sometimes seen in chromophobe adenoma and, for practical purposes, in no other tumour.

PITUITARY METASTASES

An isolated secondary deposit in the pituitary fossa is exceedingly rare, but the author has seen one case from a primary carcinoma of the colon which itself seldom gives rise to distant bone metastases. When the pituitary fossa is involved it is usually in association with multiple skeletal deposits, often from cancer of the breast. Bronchogenic carcinoma, which is the most common cause of cerebral metastases, is second in frequency, followed by the kidneys, colon and malignant tumours elsewhere. Although the destructive changes are usually evident radiologically, Mahmoud (1958) has illustrated two examples of metastases in the pituitary fossa which are hardly noticeable on the skull radiographs.

GRANULOMA

The main granulomatous lesions which may affect the pituitary hypothalamic area are; tuberculosis, sarcoidosis, histiocytosis, meningovascular syphilis and cryptococcus neoformans (Torula meningitis). However, involvement in coccidioidomycosis, histoplasmosis, blastomycosis, sporotricosis, candidiasis and aspergillosis has been mentioned by Martens and Schimrigk (1974). All these diseases are rare, but a few words about some of the more common lesions are justified.

Tuberculosis

Tuberculomas are probably the most frequent intracranial lesions in some countries where tuberculosis is still a common disease (Castro and Lepe, 1963; Tandon and Pathak, 1973). They may be single or multiple and are more frequent in the posterior fossa. In the Western hemisphere, the form which is more likely to be seen is tuberculous meningitis, sometimes leading to hydrocephalus. The skull radiographs taken many years after the disease, often show multiple small calcified tuberculomas in the basal cisterns above the pituitary fossa (Figure 5.10). Some of these patients may develop hypopituitarism due to damage to the pituitary–hypothalamic connections and pressure of the dilated third ventricle on the pituitary gland. Large solitary suprasellar tuberculomas are exceedingly rare, but one such case (Figure 2.19) has been reported (Banna, Hankinson and Odoris, 1973). Despite the rarity of the disease the possibility of tuberculoma should always be considered in the differential diagnosis of intracranial space-occupying lesions in tuberculous patients.

Sarcoidosis

Sarcoidosis affects the nervous system in 1 to 5 per cent of cases and the lesions may involve: (1) the cranial nerves, the facial being the most common, followed in decreasing order of frequency by the optic, glossopharyngeal, vagus and other nerves; (2) the spinal nerves; (3) the meninges; and (4) the brain and the spinal cord (Goodson, 1960). Intracranially the most frequent site of involvement is the base of the brain, in the form of granulomatous or adhesive arachnoiditis, or an invasion of the floor of the third ventricle. Macroscopically the lesions may be too small to be visible or rarely they may occur as a circumscribed large tumour. Common sequelae of basal involvement are optic atrophy, compression of other cranial nerves, obstructive hydrocephalus and pituitary–hypothalamic disturbances. Colover (1948) collected 20 cases from the literature with symptoms of hypothalamic dysfunction, such as diabetes insipidus, amenorrhoea, hypersomnia, lethargy, obesity and hypogonadism. Bitemporal hemianopia and enlargement of the pituitary fossa were also seen among these cases. In a more recent review of sarcoidosis of the nervous system, Schubert et al (1971) listed the incidence in various sites as follows: hypophysis and thalamus 14 per cent, other cerebral sites 41 per cent, meninges 21 per cent, optic nerves 17 per cent and spinal cord 7 per cent. Sarcoidosis seldom declares itself first in the central nervous system, but like tuberculosis, the possibility should be considered in patients with other manifestations of the disease (Silverstein, Feuer and Siltzbach, 1965; Lawrence et al, 1974).

Histiocytosis

The disease entity known as histiocytosis-X includes eosinophilic granuloma, Hand–Schüller–Christian disease and Letterer–Siwe disease. The basic disorder in these

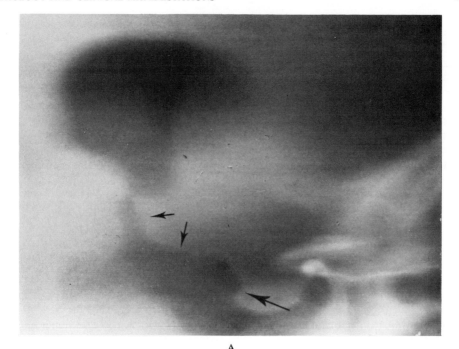

A

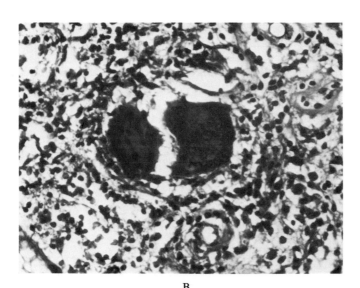

B

Figure 2.19. Massive suprasellar tuberculoma. A. Air ventriculogram (sagittal plane tomogram). There is a large filling defect in both frontal horns and a shallow defect in the anterior wall of the third ventricle (two small arrows). The anterior recesses are dilated and displaced downwards (lower arrow). B. Photomicrograph (H and E). Multiple epithelioid cells, lymphocytes, plasma cells and Langhan's giant cells are present. (By kind permission of the editor of the *British Journal of Radiology*.)

conditions is probably related and consists of idiopathic proliferation of histiocytes in children or young adults. The clinical signs vary from an isolated benign osteolytic lesion, usually affecting the skull, spine or pelvis in eosinophilic granuloma, to the malignant and fatal generalised proliferation of the reticulo-endothelial cells in Letterer–Siwe disease. Diabetes insipidus is common and may be the earliest manifestation of the disease. It is believed to be secondary to involvement of the hypothalamus, but in the majority of cases no lesion has been demonstrated. More recently a few cases have been reported in which histiocytoma of the hypothalamus, without bone involvement, was shown radiologically (Pressman, Waldron and Wood, 1975). There are no specific features, short of biopsy, which distinguish such a lesion from a hypothalamic glioma. Other manifestations of histiocytosis-X may not be apparent at the time of investigation. This is a point which should be considered if irradiation without histological verification of what appears to be a hypothalamic glioma is contemplated in a child. Radiation therapy is of little value in the visceral lesions of histiocytosis-X, particularly those of the central nervous system including the pituitary gland.

Cryptococcosis (Torulosis)

Among all fungal infections *Cryptococcus neoformans* is known for its predilection for the central nervous system. The organism has been cultured from the skin and mucous membrane of normal healthy individuals and has been isolated from the soil; it is also frequently associated saprophytically with pigeon droppings (Wilson and Plunkett, 1965). Man and animal must frequently acquire the fungi by inhalation but the disease is rare in healthy individuals, who seem to have a natural ability to resist the infection. Only when the natural resistance is diminished is man liable to acquire the disease. This is more likely to occur in association with diabetes mellitus, leukaemia, Hodgkin's disease, agammaglobulinaemia and chronic liver or respiratory disease. Torulosis is also much more common in patients who are on long-term corticosteroid treatment.

The symptoms and signs of cryptococcal invasion of the nervous system are usually referable to chronic meningitis and raised intracranial pressure, as in tuberculous meningitis. Of special importance, however, is the tendency for this disease to be accompanied by only a mild degree of inflammation while one or more large space occupying granulomas develop. This is more apt to occur in relation to the base of the brain (Swanson and Smith, 1944) and the clinical manifestations may closely simulate a neoplasm. Not infrequently, the diagnosis of cryptococcosis has been made by surgery directed toward the removal of an intracranial tumour (Wilson and Plunkett, 1965).

In conclusion it should be mentioned that meningeal inflammatory conditions may cause hypopituitarism secondary to vascular damage or a severe degree of ventricular dilatation and compression of a ballooned third ventricle upon the pituitary gland. Very occasionally a chronic granuloma is formed in the base of the brain which may then present as a suprasellar mass.

PITUITARY ABSCESS

This is uncommon in the era of antibiotics; probably no more than 20 cases having been reported (Obrador and Blazquez, 1972; Lindholm, Rasmussen and Korsgaard, 1973). Most cases occur in association with chromophobe adenoma or craniopharyngioma and are diagnosed as such prior to surgery. Predisposing conditions include chronic infections of the sphenoid sinus, sphenoid sinus pyocele (infected mucocele), cerebrospinal fluid rhinorrhoea, recurrent meningitis and thinning of the floor of the pituitary fossa from any cause.

REFERENCES

Addy, D. P. & Hudson, F. P. (1972) Diencephalic syndrome of infantile emaciation: analysis of the literature and report of further 3 cases. *Archives of Disease in Childhood*, **47**, 338–343.

Adriano, H. C. & Al-Mondhiry, H. A. B. (1967) Hemorrhagic necrosis in pituitary tumours (pituitary apoplexy). *New York State Journal of Medicine*, **67**, 1448–1452.

Adson, A. W., Kernohan, J. W. & Woltman, H. W. (1935) Cranial and Cervical Chordonas. *Archives of Neurology and Psychiatry*, **33**, 247–261.

Alexander, L. (1975) Personal Communication to D. E. Evered.

Azar-Kia, B., Krishnan, U. R. & Schecter, M. M. (1975) Neonatal craniopharyngioma. *Journal of Neurosurgery*, **42**, 91–93.

Bailey, J. A. (1973) *Disproportionate Short Stature: Diagnosis and Management*. Philadelphia, London, Toronto: W. B. Saunders.

Bailey, O. T. & Cutler, E. C. (1940) Malignant adenomas of the chromophobe cells of the pituitary body. *Archives of Pathology*, **29**, 368–399.

Banna, M. (1973) *Comprehensive study of craniopharyngioma*. MD Thesis, Newcastle Upon Tyne.

Banna, M. (1976) Craniopharyngioma: A review article based on 160 cases. *British Journal of Radiology*, **49**, 206–223.

Banna, M. (1976) Intracranial cholestatoma. *Clinical Radiology*, in press.

Banna, M. & Appleby, A. (1969) Some observations on the angiography of supratentorial meningiomas. *Clinical Radiology*, **20**, 375–386.

Banna, M., Hankinson, J. & Odoris, B. J. (1973) Interhemispheric suprasellar tuberculoma. *British Journal of Radiology*, **46**, 550–553.

Bastenie, P. A. (1946) Guérison d'un diabète acromégalique par accident vasculaire dans l'adénome hypophysaire. *Acta Clinica Beligica*, **1**, 63–71.

Becker, L. E., Yates, A. J., Hoffman, H. J. & Norman, M. G. (1975) Intracranial chordoma in infancy. *Journal of Neurosurgery*, **42**, 349–352.

Benjamin, J. E. (1929) Pituitary tumour with fulminating symptoms. *Journal of the American Medical Association*, **92**, 1755–1758.

Bergland, R. M. (1965) New information concerning the Irish giant. *Journal of Neurosurgery*, **23**, 265–269.

Bickerstaff, E. R., Small, J. M. & Guest, I. A. (1958) The relapsing course of meningioma in relation to pregnancy and menstruation. *Journal of Neurology, Neurosurgery and Psychiatry*, **21**, 89–91.

Binder, C. & Hall, P. E. (1972) *Cushing's Syndrome: Diagnosis and Management*. London: William Heinemann.

Blackwood, W. (1965) The treatment of pituitary tumours. *Proceedings of the Royal Society of Medicine*, **58**, 480–482.

Bleibtreu, L. (1905) Ein Fall von Akromegalie (Zerstörung der Hypophysis Durch Blutung). *Munchener Medizinische Wochenschrift*, **52**, 2079.

Boyce, R. & Beadles, C. F. (1893) Cited by Kobrine and Ross. A further contribution to the study of the pathology of the hypophysis cerebri. *Journal of Pathology and Bacteriology*, **1**, 359–383.

Brasel, J. A., Wright, J. C., Wilkins, L. & Bizzard, R. M. (1965) An evaluation of seventy-five patients with hypopituitarism beginning in childhood. *American Journal of Medicine*, **38**, 484–498.

British Medical Journal (1974) Assessment and management of acromegaly. *British Medical Journal*, **iv**, 549–550.

Brougham, M., Heusner, A. P. & Adams, R. D. (1950) Acute degenerative changes in adenomas of the pituitary body – with special reference to pituitary apoplexy. *Journal of Neurosurgery*, **7**, 421–439.

Cairns, H. (1938) Peripheral ocular palsies from the neurosurgical point of view. *Transactions of the Ophthalmological Society, U.K.*, **58**, 464–482.

Cartlidge, N. E. F. & Shaw, D. A. (1972) Intrasellar aneurysm with subarachnoid haemorrhage and hypopituitarism. *Journal of Neurosurgery*, **36**, 640–643.

Castro, M. & Lepe, A. (1963) Cerebral tuberculoma. *Acta Radiologica*, **i**, 821–827.

Cohen, D. N., Steinberg, M. & Buchwald, R. (1974) Suprasellar germinoma: Diagnostic confusion with optic gliomas. *Journal of Neurosurgery*, **41**, 490–493.

Colover, J. (1948) Sarcoidosis with involvement of the nervous system. *Brain*, **71**, 451–475.

Cooper, P. R. & Ransohoff, J. (1972) Craniopharyngioma originating in the sphenoid bone. *Journal of Neurosurgery*, **36**, 102–106.

Coxon, R. V. (1943) A case of haemorrhage into a pituitary tumour simulating rupture of intracranial aneurysm. *Guy's Hospital Reports*, **92**, 89–93.

Cushing, H. (1909) The hypophysis cerebri: clinical aspects of hyperpituitarism and hypopituitarism. *Journal of the American Medical Association*, **53**, 249–255.

Cushing, H. (1922) The meningiomas (dural endotheliomas): their source and favoured seats of origin. *Brain*, **45**, 282–316.

Cushing, H. (1933) 'Dyspituitarism': Twenty years later with special consideration of the pituitary adenomas. *Archives of Internal Medicine,* **51,** 487–557.

Cushing, H. & Eisenhardt, L. (1938) *Meningiomas.* Springfield, Illinois: Charles C. Thomas.

Dahlin, D. C. & MacCarty, C. S. (1952) Chordoma. A study of 59 cases. *Cancer,* **5,** 1170–1178.

Daniel, P. M., Prichard, M. M. & Schurr, P. H. (1958) Extent of the infarct in the anterior lobe of the human pituitary gland after stalk section. *Lancet,* i, 1101–1103.

Danziger, J. & Bloch, S. (1974) Hypothalamic tumours presenting as the diencephalic syndrome. *Clinical Radiology,* **25,** 153–156.

David, M. Philippon, D. & Bernard-Weil, E. (1969) The hemorrhagic forms of pituitary adenomas, etiology and clinical findings. *Presse Médicale,* **77,** 1887–1889.

Dingley, L. A. (1932) Sudden death due to a tumour of pituitary gland, *Lancet,* ii, 183–184.

Dodge, H. W. Jr, Love, J. G., Craig, W. Mck., Dockerty, M. B., Kearns, T. P., Holman, C. B. & Hayles, A. B. (1958) Gliomas of the optic nerves AMA. *Archives of Neurology and Psychiatry,* **79,** 607–621.

Doron, Y., Behar, A. & Beller, A. J. (1965) Granular cell 'myeloblastoma' of the neurohypophysis. *Journal of Neurosurgery,* **22,** 95–99.

Dott, N. M., Bailey, P. & Cushing, H. (1925) A consideration of hypophysical adenomata. *British Journal of Surgery,* **13,** 314–366.

Forbes, A. P., Henneman, P. H., Gariswold, G. C. & Abright, F. (1954) Syndrome characterised by galactorrhea, amenorrhea and low urinary FSH: comparison with acromegaly and normal lactation. *Journal of Clinical Endocrinology and Metabolism,* **14,** 265–271.

Garrison, F. H. (1929) *An Introduction to the History of Medicine,* 4th edition. Philadelphia: W. B. Saunders.

Gebel, P. (1962) Pituitary apoplexy. *Military Medicine,* **127,** 753–760.

Ghatak, N. R., Hirano, A. & Zimmerman, H. M. (1969) Intrasellar germinomas: a form of ectopic pinealoma. *Journal of Neurosurgery,* **31,** 670–675.

Girwood, T. G. & Ross, E. M. (1969) The diencephalic syndrome of early infancy. *British Journal of Radiology,* **42,** 847–850.

Givner, I. (1945) Ophthalmologic features of intracranial chordoma and allied tumours of the clivus. *Archives of Ophthalmology,* **33,** 397–403.

Glass, B. & Abbott, K. H. (1955) Subarachnoid hemorrhage consequent to intracranial tumours. *Archives of Neurology and Psychiatry,* **73,** 369–379.

Goodson, W. H. (1960) Neurologic manifestations of sarcoidosis. *Southern Medical Journal,* **53,** 1111–1116.

Gordon, D. A., Hill, F. M. & Ezrin, C. (1962) Acromegaly: a review of 100 cases. *Canadian Medical Association Journal,* **87,** 1106–1109.

Guarnaschelli, J. J. & Talalla, A. (1972) Pituitary apoplexy: a case report. *Bulletin of the Los Angeles Neurological Society,* **37,** 12–18.

Hardy, J., Robert, F., Somma, M. & Vezina, J. L. (1973) Acromegaly–gigantism: surgical treatment by transsphenoidal exeresis of the pituitary adenoma, *Neuro-chirurgie,* **19,** Supplement 2.

Henderson, J. W. (1973) *Orbital Tumours,* p. 508. Philadelphia, London, Toronto: W. B. Saunders.

Henderson, W. R. (1939) The pituitary adenomata. A follow-up study of the surgical results in 338 cases. *British Journal of Surgery,* **26,** 811–921.

Houston, J. C., Joiner, C. L. & Trounce, J. R. (1972) *A Short Textbook of Medicine.* London: The English Universities Press.

Hoyt, W. F., & Baghdassarian, S. A. (1969) Optic glioma of childhood. *British Journal of Ophthalmology,* **53,** 793–798.

Hoyt, W. F., Meshel, L. G., Lessell, S., Schatz, J. J. & Suckling, R. D. (1973) Malignant optic glioma of adulthood. *Brain,* **96,** 121–132.

Iyer, C. G. S. (1952) Case report of an adamantinoma present at birth. *Journal of Neurosurgery,* **9,** 221–228.

Jefferson, G. (1940) Extrasellar extension of pituitary adenomas. *Proceedings of the Royal Society of Medicine,* **33,** 433–458.

Jolley, F. L. & Mabon, R. L. (1958) Pituitary apoplexy. *Journal of the Medical Association of Georgia,* **47,** 75–78.

Kageyama, N. & Belsky, R. (1961) Ectopic pinealoma in the chiasmal region. *Neurology,* **11,** 318–327.

Kay, S., Lees, J. K. & Stout, A. P. (1950) Pituitary chromophete tumours of the nasal cavity. *Cancer,* **3,** 695–704.

Kirshbaum, J. D. & Chapman, B. M. (1948) Subarachnoid hemorrhage secondary to a tumour of the hypophysis with acromegaly. *Annals of Internal Medicine,* **29,** 536–540.

Kobrine, A. I. & Ross, E. (1973) Granular cell myoblastomas of the pituitary region. *Surgical Neurology,* **1,** 275–279.

Kraus, J. E. (1945) Neoplastic diseases of the human hypophysis. *Archives of Pathology,* **39,** 343–349.

Krueger, E. G., Unger, S. M. & Roswit, B. (1960) Hemorrhage into pituitary adenoma with spontaneous recovery and re-ossification of sella turcica. *Neurology,* **10,** 691–696.

Ladekarl, S. (1964) Von Recklinghausen's glioma of the optic nerve and chiasm. *Acta Ophthalmologica,* **42,** 127–138.

Lawrence, W. P., El-Gammal, T., Pool, Jr, W. H. & Apter, L. (1974) Radiological manifestations of neurosarcoidosis: report of three cases and review of literature. *Clinical Radiology,* **25,** 343–348.

Lindholm, J., Rasmussen, P. & Korsgaard, O. (1973) Intrasellar or pituitary abscess. *Journal of Neurosurgery,* **38,** 616–619.

Lippman, H. H., Onofrio, B. M. & Baker, H. L. (1971) Intrasellar aneurysm and pituitary adenoma – report of a case. *Proceedings of the Mayo Clinic,* **46,** 532–535.

List, C. F., Williams, J. R. & Balyeat, G. W. (1952) Vascular lesions in pituitary adenomas. *Journal of Neurosurgery,* **9,** 177–187.

Locke, S. & Tyler, H. R. (1961) Pituitary apoplexy. *American Journal of Medicine,* **30,** 643–648.

Long, E. R. (1927) Adenoma of hypophysis without acromegaly, hypopituitarism or visual disturbances, terminating in sudden death. *Archives of Neurology and Psychiatry,* **18,** 576–584.

Mahmoud, M. El-S. (1958) The sella in health and disease. *British Journal of Radiology,* Supplement 8, 35–37.

Males, J. L. & Townsend, J. L. (1972) Acromegaly: an analysis of twenty cases. *Southern Medical Journal,* **65,** 321–324.

Marshall, D. (1954) Glioma of the optic nerve. *American Journal of Ophthalmology,* **37,** 15–36.

Martens, H. G. & Schimrigk, K. (1974) Differential diagnosis of intracranial space-occupying lesions. *Handbook of Clinical Neurology,* Vol. 16, pp. 229–230. Amsterdam: North-Holland Publishing Company.

Mathews, W. & Wilson, C. B. (1974) Ectopic intrasellar chordoma. *Journal of Neurosurgery,* **39,** 260–263.

Matson, D. D. (1969) *Neurosurgery of Infancy and Childhood.* Springfield, Illinois: Charles C. Thomas.

McLachlan, M. S. F. & Wright, A. D. (1970) Plain film and tomographic assessment of the pituitary fossa in 140 acromegalic patients. *British Journal of Radiology,* **43,** 360–369.

Meadows, S. P. (1968) *Neuro-ophthalmology* (Ed.) Lawton Smith, J. Vol. 4, pp. 178–179. St Louis: C. V. Mosby.

Monro, J. D. R. (1913) Case of sudden death; tumour of pituitary body. *Lancet,* **ii,** 1539.

Müller, J. (1838) *Uber den Feinen Bau und die Formen der Krankhafton gescha ulster.* Berlin: Reiner.

Müller, W. & Pia, H. W. (1953) Zur klinik und Atiologie der Massenblutungen in Hypophysenadenome. *Deutsche Zeitschrift für Nervenheilkunde,* **170,** 326–336.

Nelson, D. H., Meakin, J. W. & Dealy, J. B. (1958) ACTH producing tumour of the pituitary gland. *New England Journal of Medicine,* **259,** 161–164.

Nocenti, M. R. (1968) In *Medical Physiology,* 12th edition, pp. 962–991. St Louis: C. V. Mosby.

Northfield, D. W. C. & Russell, D. S. (1967) Pubertas praecox due to hypothalmic hamartoma: report of two cases surviving surgical removal of the tumour. *Journal of Neurology, Neurosurgery and Psychiatry,* **30,** 166–173.

Nourizadeh, A. R. & Pitts, F. W. (1965) Hemorrhage into pituitary adenoma during anticoagulant therapy. *Journal of the American Medical Association,* **193,** 623–625.

Obrador, S. & Blazquez, M. G. (1972) Pituitary abscess in a craniopharyngioma. A case report. *Journal of Neurosurgery,* **36,** 785–789.

Ommaya, A. K., di Chiro, G., Baldwin, M. & Pennybacker, J. B. (1968) Non-traumatic cerebrospinal fluid rhinorrhoea. *Journal of Neurology, Neurosurgery and Psychiatry,* **31,** 214–225.

Ortiz-Suarez, H. & Erickson, D. L. (1975) Pituitary adenomas of adolescents. *Journal of Neurosurgery,* **43,** 437–439.

Peiper, W. J. & Ryan, R. J. (1961) Pituitary apoplexy in a patient with acromegaly. *Annals of Internal Medicine,* **55,** 478–481.

Philippidès, E., Steimlé, R., Lobstein, A. & Chanpy, M. (1956) Necrose d'un adeome de l'hypophyse. Signs oculaires. *Revue D'oto-neuro-Ophtalmologie,* **28,** 101–103.

Pressman, D., Waldron, R. L. & Wood, E. H. (1975) Histiocytosis-X of the hypothalamus. *British Journal of Radiology,* **48,** 176–178.

Reese, A. B. (1963) *Tumours of the Eye,* 2nd edition, pp. 532–536. New York, Evanston, London: Harper & Row.

Reverchon, L., Delater, G. & Worms, G. (1923) Contributions à l'étude des lésions traumatiques de l'hypophyse, volumineux kyste hémorrhagique de cette glande consecutif à une contusion du crâne. *Revue Neurologique,* **30,** 217–225.

Rubinstein, L. J. (1972) *Tumours of the Central Nervous System.* Washington: Armed Forces Institute of Pathology.

Sage, M. R. & McAllister, V. L. (1974) Spontaneous intracranial "aerocoele" with chromophobe adeoma. *British Journal of Radiology,* **47,** 727–729.

Schnitker, M. T. & Lehnert, H. B. (1952) Apoplexy in a pituitary chromophobe adenoma. *Journal of Neurosurgery,* **9,** 210–213.

Scholz, D. A., Gastineau, C. F. & Harrison, E. G. (1962) Cushing's syndrome with malignant chromophobe tumour of the pituitary and extracranial metastasis: report of case. *Proceedings of the Mayo Clinic*, **37**, 31–42.

Schubert, J. C. F., Gullner, H. R., Fischer, M. & Kropp, R. (1971) Boecksches Sarkoid des Nervensystems. *Deutsche Medizinische Wochenschrift*, **96**, 945–950.

Schuster, G. & Westberg, G. (1967) Gliomas of the optic nerve and chiasm. *Acta Radiologica*, **6**, 221–232.

Sheline, G. E., Boldrey, E. B. & Phillips, T. L. (1964) Chromophobe adenomas of the pituitary gland. *American Journal of Roentgenology*, **92**, 160–173.

Shenkin, H. A. (1955) Relief of amblyopia in pituitary apoplexy by prompt surgical intervention. *Journal of the American Medical Association*, **159**, 1622–1624.

Shenkin, H. A. & Crowley, J. N. (1973) Hydrocephalus complicating pituitary adenoma. *Journal of Neurosurgery and Psychiatry*, **36**, 1063–1068.

Silverstein, A., Feuer, M. M. & Siltzbach, L. E. (1965) Neurologic sarcoidosis. *Archives of Neurology*, **12**, 1–11.

Slooff, A. C. J. & Slooff, J. L. (1975) Supratentorial tumours in children. In *Handbook of Clinical Neurology*, Vol. 18, pp. 343–352. Amsterdam, Oxford: North-Holland Publishing Company.

Swanson, H. S. & Smith, W. A. (1944) Torcular granuloma simulating cerebral tumour. *Archives of Neurology and Psychiatry*, **51**, 426–431.

Tandon, P. N. & Pathak, S. N. (1973) Tuberculosis of the central nervous system. In *Tropical Neurology*, pp. 37–62. London: Oxford University Press.

Traub, S. P. (1961) *Roentgenology of Intracranial Meningiomas*. Springfield, Illinois: Charles C. Thomas.

Tytus, J. S. & Pennybacker, J. (1956) Pearly tumours in relation to the central nervous system. *Journal of Neurology, Neurosurgery and Psychiatry*, **19**, 241–259.

Uihlein, A., Balfour, W. M. & Donovan, P. F. (1957) Acute hemorrhage into pituitary adenomas. *Journal of Neurosurgery*, **14**, 140–151.

van Wagenen, W. P. (1932) Haemorrhage into pituitary tumour following trauma. *Annals of Surgery*, **95**, 625–628.

Vasconcelos, A. (1923) Apoplexia em tumor hipofisario. *Journal of Medicine*, **22**, 407.

Virchow, R. (1855) Quoted by Tytus, J. S. & Pennybacker, J. In *Virchows Archiv für Pathologische Anatomie*, **8**, 371.

Walsh, F. B. & Hoyt, W. F. (1969) *Clinical Neuro-ophthalmology*, 3rd edition, pp. 2131–2134. Baltimore: Williams & Wilkins.

Walton, J. N. (1953) Subarachnoid hemorrhage of unusual atiology. *Neurology*, **3**, 517–543.

Warren, L. O. (1951) Simmond's disease following irradiation of the pituitary gland for acromegaly. *Journal of the Maine Medical Association*, **42**, 355–356.

Weinberger, L. M., Adler, F. H. & Grant, F. C. (1940) Primary pituitary adenoma and the syndrome of the cavernous sinus – a clinical and anatomic study. *Archives of Ophthalmology*, **24**, 1197–1236.

White, J. C. & Ballantine, H. T. Jr (1961) Intrasellar aneurysms simulating hypophyseal tumours. *Journal of Neurosurgery*, **18**, 34–50.

Williams, R. H. (1968) *Textbook of Endocrinology*, pp. 63–67. Philadelphia & London: W. B. Saunders.

Willis, R. A. (1962) *The Borderland of Embryology and Pathology*, 2nd edition, pp. 442–466. London: Butterworths.

Wilson, J. W. & Plunkett, O. A. (1965) *The fungous diseases of Man*. California: Berkeley University Press.

Wolman, L. (1959) Infundibuloma. *Journal of Pathology and Bacteriology*, **77**, 283–296.

Wolman, L. & Balmforth, G. V. (1963) Precocious puberty due to a hypothalamic hamartoma in a patient surviving to late middle age. *Journal of Neurology, Neurosurgery and Psychiatry*, **26**, 275–280.

Wright, A. D., Hill, D. M., Lowy, C. & Fraser, T. R. (1970) Mortality in acromegaly. *Quarterly Journal of Medicine*, **39**, 1–16.

Wright, R. L. & Ojemann, R. G. (1965) Hemorrhage into pituitary adenomata. *Archives of Neurology*, **12**, 326–331.

Xuereb, G. P., Prichard, M. M. L. & Daniel, P. M. (1954a) The arterial supply and venous drainage of the human hypophysis cerebri. *Quarterly Journal of Experimental Physiology*, **39**, 199–217.

Xuereb, G. P., Prichard, M. M. L. & Daniel, P. M. (1954b) The hypophyseal portal system of vessels in man. *Quarterly Journal of Experimental Physiology*, **39**, 219–230.

CHAPTER THREE

Physiology, Diagnosis and Long-term Endocrine Management

D. C. EVERED

HYPOTHALAMUS AND ANTERIOR PITUITARY

General

The anterior pituitary is known to secrete seven separate protein and polypeptide hormones. The function of the anterior pituitary is controlled by the hypothalamus which secretes a number of regulatory factors (termed releasing factors or releasing hormones). The releasing hormones control the release and probably also the synthesis of the anterior pituitary hormones. Seven distinct releasing factors have now been identified (although the structure of only three of these factors has been established with certainty). Four of these factors are facilitatory and three are inhibitory. Hypothalamic extracts have, however, been described with actions which are antagonistic to the known releasing factors, and it is possible that each of the anterior pituitary hormones is under dual control. The anterior pituitary hormones, their related releasing factors and their structures are shown in Table 3.1. Some controversy exists relating to the nomenclature of the releasing factors. It has

Table 3.1. Structure of anterior pituitary hormones and releasing factors.

Anterior Pituitary Hormone	Structure	Releasing Factor/ Hormone	Structure
Thyrotrophin (TSH)	Glycoprotein	Thyrotrophin-releasing hormone (TRH)	Tripeptide
Luteinising hormone (LH)	Glycoprotein	LH/FSH-RH	Decapeptide
Follicle-stimulating hormone (FSH)	Glycoprotein	LH/FSH-RH	Decapeptide
Growth hormone (GH)	Polypeptide	GH RF	?
		GH release inhibiting hormone	Tetradecapeptide
Adrenocorticotrophic hormone (ACTH)	Polypeptide	Corticotrophin releasing factor (CRF)	?
Prolactin	Polypeptide	Prolactin release inhibiting factor (PRIF)	?
Melanocyte-stimulating hormone (MSH)	2 Polypeptides α , ß-MSH	Melanocyte-stimulating hormone release inhibiting hormone	Tripeptide

59

been suggested that when a releasing factor has been identified, its structure determined and a synthetic product prepared which is shown to have identical properties to the naturally occurring compound then this factor should be designated a hormone. This suggestion, although open to serious objections on logical grounds, is being widely adopted and will, therefore, be used here. The general term releasing factors will, however, be retained for discussing these agents as a group.

The Production and Transport of the Releasing Factors and their Control

The releasing factors are probably synthesised in the hypothalamus, although the precise areas involved have not yet been identified. They pass by axonal flow, to the median eminence, where they are stored and released into the capillaries of the hypothalamic–hypophyseal portal system, to pass to the anterior pituitary. The production and release of the releasing factors is under homeostatic control and individual control systems for each releasing factor have been described. There are, however, many situations in which the releasing factors are not regulated independently and the hypothalamus plays an important part as an integrating and co-ordinating centre for many other vegetative functions including the regulation of body temperature, water and calorie balance and sexual activity. Hypothalamic functions are, therefore, modified by many environmental stimuli (physical, psychological and biochemical) the effects of which are mediated through 'higher centres'. The major factors involved in the production and transport of the releasing factors are shown in Figure 3.1. The individual releasing hormones are also

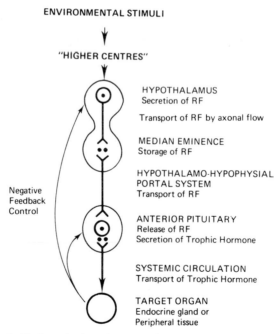

Figure 3.1. Major factors involved in the production and transport of the releasing factors.

subject to feedback control either in direct response to the metabolic effects of the anterior pituitary hormone or as a result of alteration of hormone secretion by the target endocrine gland. Individual anterior pituitary cells have been shown to be associated with the production of each of the anterior pituitary hormones in mammals and also in some cases in man. The only exception to this general rule is that ACTH and ß–MSH appear to be produced by a single anterior pituitary cell.

TRH – TSH

Thyrotrophin-releasing hormone (TRH) (Pittman, 1974)

TRH is a tripeptide, pyroglutamyl-histidyl-prolinamide. Synthetic TRH has been shown to have full biological activity in all species tested so far. TRH appears to be secreted over a wide area of the hypothalamus since lesions in the suprachiasmatic, paraventricular and arcuate-ventromedial areas have all been shown to reduce the median eminence content of TRH. There is now conclusive evidence that TRH causes the release of TSH from the pituitary and a substantial amount of indirect evidence is now available suggesting that TSH synthesis is also increased by TRH. TRH does not appear to cause the release of GH, ACTH or FSH under physiological conditions, but it does cause the release of prolactin and occasionally LH and FSH. There is some similarity between TRH and LH/FSH–RH and this may explain the latter phenomena. The explanation for the consistent release of prolactin, however, is uncertain.

Thyrotrophin (Thyroid-stimulating hormone) (TSH)

TSH is a glycoprotein hormone consisting of two subunits (designated α and ß). The α subunit is common to all the glycoprotein hormones (TSH, LH, FSH and HCG) and is necessary for full biological activity; the ß subunit is individual to each hormone and confers specificity. The release and synthesis of TSH by the anterior pituitary is under dual control (Figure 3.2). A reduced circulating thyroid hormone concentration acts directly on the hypothalamus and pituitary to stimulate TRH production and thus an increase in TSH secretion. An increased circulating thyroid hormone concentration directly inhibits TSH release from the pituitary and probably also inhibits TRH production. It seems probable that circulating thyroid hormone concentrations (thyroxine (T_4) and triiodothyronine (T_3)) in a given individual are probably maintained within rather narrow limits (Hall, Evered and Tunbridge, 1973).

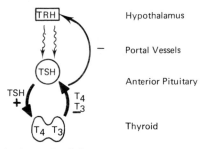

Figure 3.2. Control of TSH secretion by the anterior pituitary.

LH/FSH – RH and the Gonadotrophins

LH/FSH–RH

There is evidence in many mammals that luteinising hormone (LH) and follicle-stimulating hormone (FSH) production are under the control of separate releasing factors. The situation in man, however, appears to differ in that one hypothalamic factor has been identified – LH/FSH–RH (a decapeptide) – which consistently releases both LH and FSH, although the output of FSH in response to the exogenously administered synthetic compound is consistently less than that of LH. LH/FSH–RH does not appear to cause release of TSH, GH or ACTH (Hall, 1973).

LH and FSH

LH and FSH are both glycoprotein hormones consisting of α and ß subunits. FSH controls the development and maturation of the ovarian follicle. There is a mid-cycle peak of FSH production which probably stimulates the final rapid growth phase of the follicle. There is a sudden increase in LH secretion at mid-cycle which is associated with ovulation. LH is also necessary for the maintenance of the corpus luteum and the control of its secretory functions. FSH is responsible for the growth of the seminiferous tubules in the male, while LH controls the interstitial cells of the testis and the secretion of testosterone. LH is sometimes described as the interstitial cell stimulating hormone (ICSH) in the male. The precise mechanisms by which LH and FSH production are controlled in man are not clear at present.

Gonadotrophins in men. The serum FSH concentration remains relatively stable in man throughout the day – while serum LH levels are found to follow a circadian pattern. The serum LH concentration is low between 2 and 6 p.m. and plasma testosterone concentrations follow the fluctuations in LH concentration. There is also clear evidence that LH production is under feedback control of testosterone. Serum FSH concentrations however appear to be independent of plasma testosterone concentrations.

The factors controlling FSH secretion are less well understood. FSH levels rise with a decline in spermatogenic activity without a concomitant rise in LH, provided there is no associated lesion of the interstitial cells. The transformation of the spermatocyte II to the spermatid appears to be associated with the production of a factor which controls the secretion of FSH. It seems unlikely, on the present evidence, that this is an oestrogen. It seems probable that FSH may be controlled by a hormone (inhibin) which is secreted by the Sertoli cells, but the nature and precise functions of this suggested hormone remain obscure at present.

Gonadotrophins in women (Short, 1972). The serum FSH and LH levels are consistently high in the postmenopausal female. Oestrogen in small doses can be shown to inhibit FSH secretion, having only a small and delayed effect on LH. Larger doses of oestrogen however significantly inhibit both FSH and LH. The reverse is true of progesterone which produces marked and prolonged inhibition of LH production with a much smaller effect on FSH secretion.

The control of FSH and LH production in premenopausal women is poorly understood. There is a progressive rise in FSH production during the follicular phase and there is a peak at mid-cycle. There is a pre-ovulatory oestrogen peak which is thought to trigger the burst of LH at mid-cycle, although it is not clear at present whether this is by a positive or a negative feedback mechanism since oestrogen levels fall to very low values at ovulation.

LH then induces secretion of oestrogens and progesterone by the endocrine cells of the corpus luteum. Once the secretion of oestrogens and progesterone has been stimulated by LH then FSH and LH levels fall to very low values only to rise again toward the end of the cycle as the endocrine function of the corpus luteum fails.

It seems likely that the feedback control of gonadotrophin secretion is mediated partly indirectly through the hypothalamus and partly directly through the pituitary. It seems possible that feedback control at pituitary level assumes greater importance in man than in those species who appear to have two distinct releasing hormones.

GHRF, GH–RIH and GH

Growth hormone releasing factor (GHRF)

The structure of GHRF has not yet been determined.

Growth hormone – release inhibiting hormone (GH–RIH) (Lancet, 1974)

GH–RIH has recently been identified and found to be a tetradecapeptide. It has been shown to abolish GH release in response to hypoglycaemia and other stimuli in normal subjects and also to reduce GH levels in acromegalics. Its precise role in normal physiology has yet to be established.

Growth hormone (GH) (Raiti and Maclaren, 1974)

GH is known to consist of 188 amino acids. It is released from the pituitary in short bursts lasting from one to two hours. These episodes of GH release appear to occur most frequently at night and there are probably also long-term seasonal variations in GH secretion. A number of metabolic stimuli are known to cause GH release; these include hypoglycaemia, the administration of some amino acids (particularly arginine), fasting, malnutrition and physical exercise. Most episodes of GH secretion, however, cannot be directly related to any known stimulus to GH secretion. Hypoglycaemia, arginine and exercise are used to assess GH production clinically.

GH is known to be necessary for linear growth and the normal maturation of soft tissues. The gonadal steroids, however, are also necessary for normal skeletal maturation and pharmacological doses of glucocorticoids may interfere with the action of GH on tissues, causing impairment of growth. At least some of the actions of GH on tissues appear to be mediated by a substance known as somatomedin. GH also has other metabolic effects on protein synthesis, glucose homeostasis and fat breakdown, but it is not clear what part these actions play in normal physiology. It also has a lactogenic action.

CRF and ACTH

Corticotrophin releasing factor (CRF)

CRF has not yet been isolated and it appears to be rather more labile than the other releasing factors. Crude hypothalamic extracts can be shown to release ACTH although, inevitably, it is difficult to be certain that these effects are not due to other factors present in the extracts (e.g. vasopressin). It is well known that CRF and ACTH production and secretion vary throughout the day. The factors controlling this circadian rhythm are well recognised, although the mechanism by which their effects are mediated is poorly understood. CRF production is inhibited by cortisol and other glucocorticoids and possibly also by ACTH. CRF production is increased by a reduced circulating glucocorticoid level and by a wide range of environmental and constitutional stimuli.

Adrenocorticotrophic hormone (ACTH)

ACTH has been isolated and purified and its structure established. It is a polypeptide consisting of 39 amino acids, although only the first 24 of these seem to be necessary for biological activity. It appears that ACTH production is controlled by CRF under normal physiological conditions and all feedback control is mediated through the hypothalamus. ACTH stimulates the biosynthesis and secretion of cortisol and corticosterone. Aldosterone secretion may be transiently increased by pharmacological doses of ACTH, but this hormone appears to play no part in the normal physiological control of aldosterone secretion in most patients. ACTH can also be shown to have a melanocyte-stimulating action in man.

PRIF and Prolactin

Prolactin release inhibiting factor (PRIF)

Indirect evidence suggests that the release of prolactin by the anterior pituitary is tonically inhibited by an hypothalamic factor or factors. The disturbance of hypothalamic function by organic disease or drugs causes inappropriate lactation probably by reducing the production of PRIF. It has structural similarities to and may be identical with TRH. Recent work has shown that the TRH receptors on the thyrotroph cells have different characteristics from those on the prolactin producing cells.

Prolactin

It has now been firmly established that prolactin is an independent hormone in man. Although the complete amino-acid sequence has yet to be established it is clear that it has many structural similarities to GH. Prolactin levels are low in normal males and females. It has not been possible to identify an ovulatory prolactin peak in man although this has been identified in some mammals. It is, however, possible to show a progressive rise in serum prolactin through pregnancy and very high levels are reached at parturition. These high levels are also observed during the postpartum period and a clear response to suckling has been reported. It has also been shown that prolactin levels rise in response to stress and following administration of exogenous TRH.

The actions of prolactin are numerous, but many of the studies carried out have involved the administration of pharmacological doses of impure animal prolactin. There appears to be little doubt that prolactin plays an important role in mammary growth and lactation, although other hormones are probably also necessary for the initiation and maintenance of lactation. There is also evidence that prolactin plays a part in the maintenance of the corpus luteum, and also in the regulation of sodium and water economy. Prolactin has been reported to have a wide range of metabolic effects in animals including a synergistic action with the glucocorticoids and other metabolic actions which mimic those of GH. It remains to be established whether all these actions can be observed in man and whether they are physiological or pharmacological actions of prolactin (Forsyth and Edwards, 1972).

MRIH and MSH

Melanocyte release inhibiting hormone (MRIH)

An inhibitory factor, which has been isolated from a number of species (including man) and shown to be a tripeptide – prolyl-leucyl-glycine amide – will inhibit MSH secretion if infused in high doses. It has recently been shown that an hypothalamic peptidase can produce this substance by the degradation of oxytocin. A pentapeptide has also been described which leads to MSH release. There is considerable doubt surrounding the possible physiological role of these substances.

Melanocyte-stimulating hormone (MSH)

The pituitaries of most species can be shown to contain two melanocyte-stimulating peptides. α -MSH contains 13 amino acids and is identical with the first 13 amino acids of ACTH. ß-MSH shows considerably more species variation and is less active than α -MSH under experimental conditions. ß-MSH, however, appears to be the hormone which is actively secreted by the pituitary in man. It also bears a strong structural resemblance to ACTH. The physiological function of MSH in man is unknown, but its secretion can be shown to occur in parallel with ACTH, and MSH appears to originate from the adrenocorticotrophic cells of the anterior pituitary.

HYPOTHALAMUS AND POSTERIOR PITUITARY

General

The posterior pituitary is not a discrete endocrine gland, but merely the most distal part of an endocrine neurosecretory system which also includes various hypothalamic areas – most notably the supra-optic and paraventricular nuclei and the neurohypophyseal tract. Antidiuretic hormone (ADH or vasopressin) and oxytocin are found in much higher concentrations in the hypothalamus than at any other site in the nervous system. Oxytocin and human ADH (arginine vasopressin) are structurally very similar and each consists of eight amino acids with a 5-member S–S bonded ring and a tail consisting of three amino acids. The amino-acid sequence of these hormones differs only in two locations – one on the ring and one on the tail. Both hormones are synthesised in the hypothalamus (ADH in the supra-optic nucleus and oxytocin in the paraventricular nucleus) and then pass by axonal flow to the posterior pituitary. They pass down the neurohypophyseal tract in loose association with a carrier protein, neurophysin, which is also released with the posterior pituitary hormones into the circulation.

ADH

ADH plays a major role in the regulation of water balance, by virtue of its actions on the distal convoluted tubule and the collecting ducts. Water reabsorption is regulated by the permissive role of this hormone which, under suitable physiological conditions, allows the reabsorption of water along an established osmotic gradient. There are three major factors which regulate ADH secretion: plasma osmolality, extracellular fluid volume and body temperature. The relative importance of these factors varies in relation to environmental stimuli, but experimental work suggests that the maintenance of plasma osmolality within narrow limits is the dominant influence in a temperate climate.

Oxytocin

The role of oxytocin in normal physiology is unknown. It is clear that its major pharmacological action is causing contraction of the uterine musculature, although it also has some action on the ejection of milk and on sodium and water balance.

TESTS OF PITUITARY AND HYPOTHALAMIC FUNCTION

Pituitary and hypothalamic function may be assessed in a number of ways:
1. Assessment of pituitary function under basal conditions (i.e. direct measurement of circulating trophic hormone concentration).
2. Assessment of function of target organs (i.e. other endocrine glands or peripheral tissues).
3. Stress tests. Measurement of pituitary hormone concentrations under basal conditions will, at best, only demonstrate major disturbances of function. A stress test may be used to demonstrate the ability of the endocrine control system to adapt to homeostatic disturbances and may reveal minor degrees of impairment of function. Stimulation tests are, therefore, carried out in suspected hypofunction and suppression tests in suspected hyperfunction.

The investigation of pituitary and hypothalamic function will, therefore, be described on this basis. (Details of standard tests can be found in Hall et al, 1974.)

TSH

Suspected hypofunction

Serum TSH assay. Measurement of serum TSH concentration alone is unhelpful since low levels are seen in many normal subjects. (An elevated serum TSH concentration implies primary thyroid failure (Hall, 1972).)

Tests of thyroid function. Routine measurements of circulating thyroid hormone concentration (thyroxine, protein-bound iodine (PBI) and a T_3 resin or sephadex uptake) may be carried out. The finding of low levels of circulating thyroid hormone in the absence of an elevated serum TSH is strong presumptive evidence of failure of TSH production. Indirect evidence of failure of endogenous TSH production may also be obtained by carrying out a radio-iodine uptake before and after the administration of exogenous TSH. A significant increase in uptake, from a previously low value, following TSH stimulation suggests failure of endogenous TSH production, while an absent response implies primary thyroid failure. Difficulty may be experienced in interpreting the results of these investigations for two reasons. Firstly, conventional tests of thyroid function may lie within the accepted normal range in subjects with minor degrees of thyroid deficiency and secondly subjects with a minor degree of primary thyroid failure may show a response to TSH stimulation (Evered, 1974).

Stress test. Serum TSH concentrations may be measured following administration of TRH. Failure of the serum TSH concentration to rise following TRH in subjects with reduced thyroid function is strong presumptive evidence of failure of pituitary TSH production. Patients with hypothalamic disease will show a rise in TSH following exogenous TRH but the time course of this release is prolonged compared with normal subjects. A range of responses may however be seen in pituitary and hypothalamic disease. A normal TRH response excludes pituitary or hypothalamic abnormality whereas an absent or impaired response indicates those at risk.

It may be difficult to demonstrate or exclude a minor degree of thyroid deficiency secondary to failure of TSH production, and in cases of difficulty a therapeutic trial of thyroxine may be necessary (Hall, Evered and Tunbridge, 1973).

Suspected hyperfunction

Hyperthyroidism is only very rarely due to overproduction of TSH (Hoffenberg, 1974). A few patients have been described with pituitary tumours or hypothalamic disturbance in whom hyperthyroidism has been associated with an elevated serum TSH. The majority of patients with hyperthyroidism have no evidence of hypothalamic or pituitary disease and have a low (normal) serum TSH concentration which fails to rise after TRH.

LH and FSH

Suspected hypofunction

Measurement of gonadotrophin concentrations. Measurement of plasma or urinary gonadotrophins (LH and/or FSH) is generally adequate to distinguish between primary gonadal failure (when high levels are found) and failure secondary to pituitary or hypothalamic disease.

Tests of gonadal function. These are generally less helpful and inevitably urinary oestrogen and testosterone concentrations are reduced.

Stress tests. 1. Clomiphene (a synthetic non-steroidal compound) causes gonadotrophin release (especially of LH), possibly by acting as an anti-oestrogen at the hypothalamic level. Administration of clomiphene over five days with serial plasma or urine LH estimations can therefore be used as a stress test of the hypothalamic pituitary capacity to secrete gondadotrophins (Newton et al, 1971).

2. LH/FSH – RH may be used as a test of pituitary reserve of LH and FSH; although further studies are still required to establish the limits of normal response in relation to age, sex and the menstrual cycle. It may be possible to separate pituitary and hypothalamic causes of gonadotrophin failure using this agent and clomiphene, although many patients with pituitary tumours and amenorrhoea will respond to a pharmacological dose of LH/FSH-RH (Mortimer et al, 1973).

These tests are rarely required for diagnostic purposes in subjects with pituitary or hypothalamic disease although these agents do have considerable therapeutic value.

Growth Hormone

Suspected hypofunction

Measurement of GH concentrations. Circulating GH levels are low in many normal subjects and single measurements are therefore valueless.

Peripheral tissue function. There is no suitable test of end organ function to demonstrate

GH deficiency although it can be shown that serum levels of somatomedin are low in pituitary failure.

Stress tests. Circulating levels of GH in normal subjects rise in response to hypoglycaemia. GH deficiency may, therefore, be demonstrated by an insulin sensitivity test (0.1 U soluble insulin/kg body weight) (Greenwood, Landon and Stamp, 1966). The following responses may be seen.

Normals – rise to 20 mcg/l (20 ng/ml) or greater.

Partial failure – rise to 10–20 mcg/l (10–20 ng/ml).

Severe failure – rise to less than 10 mcg/l (10 ng/ml).

It is important when carrying out an insulin sensitivity test to:
1. Establish that an adequate hypoglycaemic stimulus has been given by measuring the blood glucose and demonstrating a fall to less than 2.0 nmol/l (40 mg/100 ml). The presence of hypoglycaemic symptoms provides useful confirmatory information.
2. Carry out the test in hospital patients, in the presence of a doctor and with parenteral glucose and hydrocortisone immediately available. If severe neuroglycopenia does occur, the test should be terminated immediately by 40 ml 50 per cent glucose intravenously followed by an infusion. Intravenous hydrocortisone should be given if the patient's symptoms do not improve rapidly with glucose.
3. Avoid the test in patients with severe pituitary failure who show an increased sensitivity to insulin. If it needs to be carried out in such patients then a smaller dose of insulin (i.e. 0.05 U/kg) should be given. This test should also be avoided in patients with angina and epilepsy.

It is possible to use other stimuli (see above) to demonstrate GH deficiency and such tests are generally considered to be more appropriate, at least in the first instance, in children, particularly if an isolated GH deficiency is suspected.
1. Exercise test. The GH level is measured before and twenty minutes after strenuous exercise on an ergometer.
2. Bovril test. Bovril (20 g/1.5m² body surface) is given by mouth in warm water and GH levels are measured before and serially for two hours after administration.

A negative response to either of the above tests must be confirmed either by an insulin sensitivity test or by an arginine test. A positive response to any of these stimuli, however, excludes GH deficiency.
3. Arginine. Arginine (0.5 g/kg body weight to a maximum of 30 g) is infused intravenously over a 30-minute period and serial samples for GH estimation are taken over the following two and a half hours. This test is of greatest value in children and women. Men may not respond adequately unless pretreated with oestrogens.

Suspected hyperfunction (British Medical Journal, 1974)

Measurement of GH Levels. Fasting levels of GH are raised, but elevated levels may be seen in many normal subjects in response to physiological stimuli. A low level, however, excludes active hypersecretion of GH (gigantism or acromegaly).

Peripheral tissue function. The peripheral tissue effects of excess growth hormone production are frequently obvious. Confirmation may be obtained by demonstrating an increased heel pad or skin thickness. Impaired carbohydrate tolerance, an increase in serum phosphate and occasionally hypercalcaemia are seen. None of these abnormalities, however, is specific.

Stress tests. 1. Glucose tolerance test (GTT). GH levels are reduced to 5mcg/l (5 ng/ml) or less during a $2\frac{1}{2}$ hour oral GTT. This test must be continued for $2\frac{1}{2}$ hours since the surges of GH secretion may last for up to 2 hours in normals. Failure of suppression demonstrates inappropriate hypersecretion of GH, thus confirming the presence of gigantism or acromegaly.

2. Augmented insulin sensitivity test. Subjects with acromegaly are more resistant to insulin than normal subjects and the degree of resistance may be assessed by serial blood glucose estimations following intravenous insulin in a dose of 0.3 U/kg body weight.

This test rarely adds anything to those already described, it is not without risk and should never be carried out if there is any clinical suspicion of hypopituitarism. A relatively large dose of insulin may be required, however, to test pituitary ACTH reserve in acromegaly.

ACTH

Suspected hypofunction

Measurement of ACTH concentration. Serum ACTH concentrations are low or in the low/normal range in pituitary ACTH failure. These estimations are technically difficult and the information can be obtained more simply by a stress test.

Adrenocortical function. The plasma levels of cortisol often lie within the lower part of the normal range in pituitary failure and are, therefore, generally unhelpful.

Stress test. Insulin-induced hypoglycaemia stresses the whole of the hypo-thalamic–pituitary–adrenal axis (Greenwood, Landon and Stamp, 1966). The plasma cortisol is measured serially during the course of a standard insulin sensitivity test (see above). No rise or a small rise following an adequate hypoglycaemic stimulus implies impaired pituitary ACTH reserve (providing adrenal function is normal). The plasma cortisol will rise to a value greater than 550 nmol/1 (20 μg/100 ml) in normal subjects.

The precautions described previously in relation to this test must be meticulously observed. It is important to demonstrate that normal adrenal responsiveness to ACTH (synacthen or tetracosactrin) exists, if there is any doubt, before these other investigations can be reliably interpreted.

Other stress tests, metyrapone test, lysine–vasopressin test and the pyrogen test are available but are rarely, if ever, of practical value. Lysine–vasopressin is said to test the pituitary ACTH-producing mechanism, but it is not now accepted that this agent acts directly or entirely on the anterior pituitary.

Suspected hyperfunction

Measurement of ACTH concentration. The measurement of serum ACTH concentration is of great value in the investigation of Cushing's syndrome. Approximately 85 per cent of patients with spontaneously occurring Cushing's syndrome develop hypercortisolism as a result of an increased pituitary ACTH production. The ACTH levels are generally in the upper part of the normal range or moderately elevated and are inappropriately high in relation to the plasma cortisol concentration. There is a loss of the normal circadian rhythm of ACTH secretion. Very high levels suggest the presence of the ectopic ACTH syndrome.

Adrenocortical function. Plasma cortisol concentrations are generally in the upper part of the normal range or only slight elevated, but the circadian rhythm is lost. Care must be taken, particularly with obese patients, since the stress of a difficult venepuncture can produce an increase in plasma cortisol concentration. The urinary excretion of 11-hydroxycorticosteroid (free cortisol) is high in Cushing's syndrome (Mattingly and Tyler, 1967).

Stress test. Occasional difficulty is encountered in patients with a depressive illness in whom Cushing's syndrome is suspected. Such subjects may have a high plasma cortisol and a high plasma ACTH as a result of depression. They can be distinguished from those with hypothalamic – pituitary dependent Cushing's syndrome by an insulin sensitivity test. Patients with depressive illnesses show a further rise in plasma cortisol in response to hypoglycaemia, whereas those with Cushing's syndrome show no response.

The dexamethasone suppression test is still used in the investigation of Cushing's syndrome. It may be misleading and is not necessary now that it is possible to measure the serum ACTH concentration directly.

Prolactin

Measurement of prolactin concentration. Serum prolactin levels are low in hypopituitarism and have been shown to be high in many subjects with galactorrhoea, particularly when this is associated with a pituitary tumour. High prolactin levels are found in a majority of patients with apparently non-functioning pituitary tumours even in the absence of galactorrhoea. High prolactin levels may also be seen in acromegaly, but it is not clear at present whether galactorrhoea in this condition is always accompanied by prolactin secretion or whether it may be due to the lactogenic activity of GH.

Peripheral tissue function. Increased prolactin secretion becomes evident clinically when galactorrhoea occurs. There is no test of peripheral tissue function which reflects an increased circulating prolactin concentration in the absence of inappropriate lactation.

Stress tests. It can be shown that serum prolactin levels rise in normal subjects, but not in those with hypopituitarism, following administration of phenothiazines and TRH. Ergot alkaloids and L-dopa suppress prolactin production. The action of L-dopa is mediated through PRIF while the ergot alkaloids act directly on the pituitary. No standard stress test of prolactin production has been established at present.

ADH

Suspected hypofunction

Measurement of ADH concentration. This estimation is technically difficult, of little value in suspected ADH deficiency and is not generally available.

Peripheral tissue test. The serum osmolality is high or high/normal in primary polyuria secondary to ADH deficiency, since the patient remains continuously moderately dehydrated, thus providing the stimulus to thirst. The reverse is true in patients with primary polydipsia (e.g. compulsive water drinking) who have a low or low/normal serum osmolality. The urine osmolality is low in both situations.

Stress test. A standard fluid deprivation test in subjects with primary polyuria will cause a further rise in the serum osmolality while the urine volume remains large and the urine osmolality low (Barlow and de Wardener, 1959). Such a response in the absence of other evident causes of primary polyuria provides presumptive evidence of endogenous ADH deficiency and this can be confirmed by the administration of an ADH preparation which will cause a rapid reduction in urine volume and a rise in urine osmolality in all cases of ADH deficiency.

THE ENDOCRINE INVESTIGATION OF SUSPECTED HYPO-THALAMIC–PITUITARY DISEASE

Hypopituitarism

Pituitary tumours may be associated with some degree of anterior pituitary failure. This is particularly true of non-functional tumours. This may be the result of pituitary compression or may follow expansion of the tumour outside the fossa compressing the stalk or hypothalamus. Frequently failure of all or several of the pituitary hormones is present although occasionally isolated deficiencies may be seen. Gonadotrophin deficiency is usually seen as the first manifestation of endocrine failure followed by GH deficiency and then ACTH and/or TSH deficiency.

A suggested plan for the assessment of suspected anterior pituitary failure is shown in Table 3.2. This provides a basic guide to investigation; other investigations may be of value in selected patients. The following points should be noted.

1. A purely clinical assessment will only reveal major deficiencies of trophic hormones. Laboratory investigation is, therefore, mandatory in all cases.
2. The precautions relating to the insulin sensitivity test must always be rigorously observed.
3. Pituitary function in patients with pituitary tumours should always be assessed before and after definitive treatment, unless complete failure is present initially. A limited assessment may be acceptable before destructive therapy to the pituitary.
4. Posterior pituitary function cannot be adequately assessed in the presence of anterior pituitary failure.

Table 3.2. Investigation of suspected anterior pituitary failure.

Clinical	Note presence or absence of following features
LH and FSH	Impotence, infertility, oligo- or amenorrhoea
GH	Child – growth failure
	Adult – nil
ACTH	Weakness, nausea, vomiting, hypoglycaemia
TSH	Child – growth retardation
	Adult – Lassitude, cold intolerance, dryness of skin, prolongation of reflexes
MSH	Pallor – failure to tan on exposure to UV light
Laboratory	
LH and FSH	Plasma and/or urine LH and FSH
GH	Insulin sensitivity test (or other stress test in child)
ACTH	Insulin sensitivity test
TSH	Serum thyroxine, TRH test and/or ^{131}I uptake before and after exogenous TSH

Acromegaly

Acromegaly is usually insidious in its onset and, therefore, the skeletal and soft tissue changes are often advanced by the time the patient presents to hospital. The change may be assessed by reviewing old photographs of the patient. Radiological assessment will usually reveal an enlarged pituitary fossa, and an increase in heel pad and skin thickness. The diagnosis, however, rests upon demonstrating an elevated serum GH concentration which fails to fall during an oral glucose tolerance test. Investigation in acromegaly should always include assessment of the function of the other anterior pituitary hormones.

Cushing's Syndrome

The generic term Cushing's syndrome is used to describe those syndromes which arise from increased circulating glucocorticoid concentrations. Cushing's syndrome may therefore be classified as in Table 3.3. It is, of course, possible to exclude ACTH or steroid administration at the outset. Investigation should then follow the lines indicated in Table 3.4.

Table 3.3. Classification of Cushing's syndrome.

ACTH dependent	ACTH independent
1. Hypothalamic-pituitary dependent (Cushing's disease)	1. Adrenal adenoma
2. Ectopic ACTH syndrome	2. Adrenal carcinoma
3. ACTH administration	3. Steroid administration

Galactorrhoea

Galactorrhoea may be defined as lactation in the absence of an appropriate physiological stimulus. The causes of galactorrhoea are summarised in Table 3.5. The investigation of the patient with galactorrhoea may present considerable difficulty. The lines of investigation are summarised in Table 3.6. Galactorrhoea following the administration of an oral contraceptive or phenothiazine is common. The exclusion of drug-induced galactorrhoea allows the remaining patients to be divided into three broad categories:
1. Galactorrhoea associated with pituitary–hypothalamic disturbance.
2. Galactorrhoea associated with other endocrine disease which is generally clinically apparent.
3. Galactorrhoea associated with a local lesion or non-endocrine disease which is generally clinically apparent.

It is the first group which may cause the greatest diagnostic difficulty since frequently a pituitary lesion cannot be demonstrated. The galactorrhoea can, however, frequently be modified by the use of drugs. Such subjects require careful follow-up since a proportion will develop a pituitary tumour at a later date.

Diabetes Insipidus

Diabetes insipidus occurs uncommonly in pituitary tumours. Simple destruction of the posterior lobe or pituitary stalk at worst only causes transient diabetes insipidus, since

Table 3.4. Investigation of suspected Cushing's syndrome.

1. Is hypercortisolism present?
   a. Plasma cortisol estimations at 9 a.m., 4 p.m. and 12 m.n. on two successive days.
   b. 24-hour urine for free cortisol (11-hydroxycorticosteroids) on two successive days.
   If 'yes' proceed to (2).
2. Is hypercortisolism ACTH dependent?
   Plasma ACTH estimations with cortisol estimations at 9 a.m., 4 p.m. and 12 m.n.
   If 'yes' proceed to (3).
   If 'no' proceed to (4).
3. Is this Cushing's disease or ectopic ACTH syndrome?
   Examine clinical and laboratory data.

	Cushing's disease	Ectopic ACTH syndrome
Progression	Slow	Rapid
Pigmentation	6%	90%
Oedema	Absent or mild	Severe
Muscle weakness	Mild	Severe
Weight loss	Absent or mild	Rapid and severe
Carbohydrate intolerance	Minor	Severe
Serum potassium	Generally normal	Low
Urine free cortisol (times normal)	2–3	2–20
Plasma ACTH	40 – 100 ng/l (40–100 pg/ml)	usually > 200 ng/l (>200pg/ml)

Then look for pituitary tumour or other primary neoplasm (e.g. bronchus) as appropriate.
(N.B. Occasionally a depressive illness will mimic Cushing's disease. An insulin sensitivity test is the best discriminant.)
4. Is this adrenal adenoma or carcinoma?
   Angiography followed by surgical exploration.

Table 3.5. Causes of galactorrhoea.

1. *Hypothalamic-pituitary disease*
   Pituitary tumours
      Otherwise non-functioning adenomata
      Cushing's disease
      Acromegaly
   Partial hypopituitarism
      Particularly after pituitary stalk section
2. *Other endocrine disease*
   Primary hypothyroidism
   Hyperthyroidism
   Oestrogen-secreting tumours
3. *Non-endocrine disease*
   Local injury or inflammatory disease of chest wall
   Prolactin production by non-endocrine tumours
   Sacroid
4. *Drugs*
   Oral contraceptives
   Phenothiazines
   Reserpine
   Methyldopa
   Tricyclic antidepressants
   Haloperidol

Table 3.6. Investigation of galactorrhoea.

---

1. Clinical
   a. Obtain a full drug history
   b. Examine for local lesion of chest wall
   c. Note signs of overt endocrine disease
2. Pituitary function
   a. Appropriate tests for Cushing's disease, acromegaly and partial hypopituitarism
   b. Skull x-ray
3. Thyroid function
   a. Serum TSH estimation
   b. Serum thyroxine concentration
4. Miscellaneous
   Chest x-ray

ADH is still able to escape into the systemic circulation from the axons of the hypothalamic neurones. A lesion has to be sufficiently large to produce considerable destruction of the hypothalamus before diabetes insipidus occurs. Diabetes insipidus occurs much more frequently after pituitary surgery or following a pituitary implant (e.g. ^{90}Y); the diabetes insipidus may then be transient or permanent.

Diabetes insipidus may not be apparent in subjects with anterior pituitary failure since adequate circulating glucocorticoid concentrations are necessary to clear a water load, and this must clearly be borne in mind when investigating pituitary function.

The patient who presents with polydipsia and polyuria may be suffering from either primary polydipsia (e.g. compulsive water drinking) with secondary polyuria or primary polyuria (e.g. ADH deficiency) with secondary polydipsia. The investigation of polydipsia and polyuria should follow the lines indicated in Table 3.7.

LONG-TERM ENDOCRINE MANAGEMENT

Pituitary tumours may be associated with some degree of anterior pituitary failure. This is particularly true of 'non-functional' tumours. Endocrine failure may be the result of pituitary compression or may follow expansion of the tumour outside the fossa compressing the stalk or hypothalamus. Frequently failure of all or several of the pituitary

Table 3.7. Investigation of suspected diabetes insipidus.

---

1. Does the patient have polydipsia and polyuria?
   Admit to hospital
   Fluid intake and output recorded under strict supervision
   If yes (fluid throughput $>$ 2.5l/24 hours) proceed to 2
2. Is this primary polydipsia or primary polyuria?
   Serum osmolality
   Fluid deprivation test under close supervision with regular weighing of patient
   If primary polydipsia – proceed to 3
   If primary polyuria – proceed to 4
3. Primary polydipsia – Cause?
   Most commonly due to compulsive water drinking
   Exclude hypercalcaemia, hypokalaemia and hyperthyroidism by appropriate tests
4. Primary polyuria – Cause?
   Exclude osmotic and renal causes by appropriate tests
   Response to endogenous ADH

---

hormones is present, although occasionally isolated deficiencies may be seen. Gonadotrophin deficiency is usually seen as the first manifestation of endocrine failure followed by GH deficiency and then ACTH and/or TSH deficiency. It is important to assess pituitary function before and after definitive treatment — unless complete failure is present initially. Endocrine replacement therapy should only be started in subjects with biochemically proven trophic hormone deficiency.

ACTH Deficiency

Failure of ACTH secretion may be complete, so that cortisol levels are reduced even under basal conditions, or partial with diminished cortisol production only being apparent under conditions of stress. Replacement therapy with glucocorticoids is, of course, mandatory in subjects with reduced cortisol levels under basal conditions, and is generally desirable in those with partial failure of ACTH production. The latter subjects have an inadequate response to stress and their increased cortisol requirements in the event of trauma, illness or surgery are more likely to be recognised if they are already on replacement therapy and carrying a 'steroid' card.

Maintenance therapy generally consists of cortisol 20 to 30 mg daily in divided doses. It is usual practice to give 20 mg in the morning and 10 mg in the evening to mimic the normal circadian rhythm of cortisol secretion. Plasma cortisol levels are, however, very variable in subjects on replacement therapy and thus the cortisol levels should be checked in patients taking their usual substitution therapy. Blood samples are taken before and then 30 and 60 minutes after the morning dose of cortisol and thereafter every 2 hours until the evening dose is due. The peak level is usually reached within 60 min and the dose should be adjusted to give a peak value of around 800 nmol/l (30 μg/100 ml) and a level which does not fall below 120 nmol/l (4 μg/100 ml) just before the next dose is due. It may be necessary to give the dose three or even four times daily in view of the rather short pharmacological half-life of cortisol. Assessment cannot be carried out adequately while subjects are receiving oestrogen replacement therapy since these steroids lead to an increase in transcortin concentration and thus the total plasma cortisol concentration is misleading. Mineralocorticoid replacement is not required.

It is important to instruct patients to carry a card or to wear a bracelet at all times stating that they are receiving glucocorticoid replacement therapy. The dose must be increased in the event of illness, trauma or surgery and the increase in dose should be related to the severity of the stress. Cortisol sodium succinate (100 mg) can be given intravenously and repeated as necessary for acute stress. During the recovery phase from surgery or trauma intramuscular cortisone acetate (50 to 100 mg), which has a longer half-life may be used. Clearly the steroid requirements in times of stress must be assessed on an individual, if rather arbitrary, basis.

TSH Deficiency

Thyroid failure should be treated with thyroxine. The initial dose should not exceed 0.05 mg daily in patients over 40 years of age; an initial dose of 0.1 mg daily may be used in younger patients. The dose should be increased by 0.05 mg increments until the patient is euthyroid. Recent work has shown that conventional replacement therapy with 0.3 mg daily is almost invariably excessive and that the euthyroid state is maintained by 0.1 to 0.2 mg daily. It is important that any associated ACTH deficiency is treated before the TSH deficiency, since thyroxine can precipitate acute adrenocortical insufficiency in the ACTH deficient subjects.

Gonadotrophin Deficiency

Females

Cyclical therapy. Cyclical hormone therapy should be introduced in the female under the age of 45. The aim of cyclical therapy is to produce or maintain normal feminisation, to defer, if possible, those degenerative changes which may follow the premature cessation of menstruation, and to induce the psychological benefits of regular menstruation – even if this is only due to oestrogen withdrawal. Regular withdrawal bleeding is most easily achieved if a progestational agent is used in addition to an oestrogen. This may be suitably achieved by the administration of ethinyloestradiol in a dose of 0.01 mg twice daily for 24 days and adding norethisterone, 5 mg daily, for the last ten days of the course. The discontinuation of therapy is usually followed by withdrawal bleeding and a further course of cyclical therapy may be introduced after the bleeding has ceased. Bleeding may not occur for the first one or two cycles and then therapy is restarted after an interval of six or seven days. (It is frequently convenient to start each cycle on the first day of each calendar month.) It is sometimes necessary to increase the dose of oestrogen to achieve regular withdrawal bleeding. It is, of course, possible to establish regular menstrual bleeding by use of one of the many oral contraceptive preparations available. The therapeutic regimen recommended above does, however, have two major advantages. It allows much more flexibility in dosage and it is generally possible to use a much lower dose of oestrogen than is present in even the 'low oestrogen' oral contraceptive preparations. Care must be taken in adolescent patients before epiphyseal fusion, particularly if there is an associated GH deficiency, to avoid premature cessation of growth. It is usually, therefore, desirable to delay cyclical therapy in such patients for as long as possible, or until an adequate height is achieved.

Infertility. Infertility in the female may follow any disturbance of normal hypothalamic–pituitary function. The treatment of infertility in such patients should usually be carried out by a specialist clinic. It is possible to induce ovulation in subjects with pituitary failure by treatment with FSH and HCG. There is general agreement that an FSH preparation which contains some LH activity is needed and human menopausal gonadotrophin (HMG – Pergonal) is a convenient preparation. The total dose is divided into three equal injections given over a period of five days and followed on the eighth day by HCG (5000 IU). The total dose of FSH is increased each month until ovulation occurs, as shown by an increase in urinary oestrogens and, later, pregnanediol. It is important to regulate the total FSH dosage carefully and only increase the dose by small increments. Appropriate supervision will generally make it possible to avoid the problems of multiple ovulation, and the 'hyper-stimulation syndrome'. Meticulous antenatal care is, of course mandatory following conception.

Clomiphene is ineffective in women with organic hypopituitarism.

Males

Androgen therapy. Androgen replacement therapy is indicated in all subjects with reduced Leydig cell function secondary to gonadotrophin deficiency. A number of testosterone preparations and analogues are available and are listed in Table 3.8. Those preparations which are generally most suitable in practice are marked with an asterisk. Methyl testosterone preparations should not be used since there is a risk of inducing cholestatic jaundice with these agents. Adequate replacement therapy is indicated by the

Table 3.8. Androgen preparations.

Preparation	Route	Dose	Dose schedule
Testosterone propionate*	Sublingual	10 mg	3 or 4 times daily
Fluoxymesterone	Oral	5 mg	1 to 3 times daily
Mesterolone	Oral	25 mg	2 to 4 times daily
Testosterone esters in oil (Sustanon - 250)*	IM	250 mg	1 or 2 times monthly
Testosterone oenathate in oil	IM	250 mg	1 or 2 times monthly
Testosterone implants*	SC	100 mg	3 to 6 pellets SC every 4 to 6 months

* See text.

development of secondary sexual characteristics, libido and normal potency. Overdosage is rare and is usually indicated by over-frequent erections and excessive sebum secretion.

Infertility. It is rarely possible to treat infertility which is associated with anterior pituitary failure successfully. The response to gonadotrophin preparations (e.g. Pergonal, which is derived from human menopausal urine and is rich in FSH but also contains some LH), is variable and is related in part to the duration of failure of gonadotrophin production. Therapy must be prolonged, since spermatozoa take about three months to mature and successes are rare. LH/FSH–RH has been reported to be successful in inducing spermatogenesis in occasional patients with pituitary disease, but more extensive studies are required before the therapeutic role of this agent can be established.

GH Deficiency

GH deficiency in the adult does not require replacement therapy. Deficiency in the child does, however, require treatment and is usually successful if the patient's bone age is less than 14 years. Human GH is required and the supply and distribution of this hormone in the UK is controlled by the MRC. The following criteria must be fulfilled to obtain a supply of GH:
1. The child must be below the third percentile for height.
2. The lack of linear growth must have been documented for at least a year.
3. The child must show a lack of GH production during an appropriate stress test.
4. The child must be receiving adequate replacement therapy with other hormones if this is necessary.
Treatment is given by intramuscular injection (10 mg twice weekly) and this should be continued until adequate growth has been achieved. Clearly replacement with gonadal hormones must be withheld until growth is adequate.

ADH Deficiency

Vasopressin. The standard treatment of diabetes insipidus for many years has been vasopressin. Aqueous vasopressin has a short duration of action (one to two hours) but may be of value in controlling the transient diabetes insipidus which sometimes follows surgery to the pituitary.

Vasopressin tannate in oil has a longer duration of action (24 to 48 hours) and is administered by intramuscular injection. It is important to take considerable care over the injection technique. The ampoule must be warmed to 35°C before drawing the suspension into the syringe to ensure that all the vasopressin is adequately suspended in the oil. The injection site must be varied to avoid the accumulation of depots of oil which will otherwise interfere with absorption. The dose must be adjusted for each individual but is generally between 2 to 4 IU every 1 to 2 days.

Lysine vasopressin (50 IU/ml) is available as a nasal spray and is of value in some patients although resistance may develop. The dose can be simply adjusted to the patient's requirements by advising him to spray once into each nostril at each act of micturition and twice into each nostril before retiring.

Desamino-D-arginine vasopressin (DDAVP) is a vasopressin analogue which is potent and well absorbed by the nasal route. This agent is now the most satisfactory treatment for diabetes insipidus.

Oral agents. Chlorpropamide, the oral hypoglycaemic agent (a sulphonylurea), has recently been shown to reduce free water clearance in subjects with central diabetes insipidus. Experimental work suggests that this agent increases the tissue sensitivity to small quantities of ADH. Chlorpropamide may therefore be useful in partial diabetes insipidus or in reducing the requirements for exogenous vasopressin preparations. Care must be exercised when using chlorpropamide to avoid hypoglycaemia – and also the other adverse effects of this drug must be borne in mind (skin rashes, gastrointestinal disturbance and blood dyscrasias).

Other oral agents include the thiazides, and other natriuretic diuretics whose action is probably related to sodium depletion and carbamazepine and clofibrate which may have an action similar to that of chlorpropamide. None of these agents plays a part in the routine treatment of diabetes insipidus at the present time.

Summary

Replacement therapy is generally best carried out with vasopressin preparations (DDAVP is most satisfactory). The nasal preparations are convenient but occasionally resistance may develop and a parenteral preparation may be required. Chlorpropamide is occasionally of value alone in partial diabetes insipidus, but fatalities have occurred due to hypoglycaemia since this drug has a long half-life and its routine use cannot be recommended.

REFERENCES

Barlow, E. D. & de Wardener, H. E. (1959) Compulsive water drinking. *Quarterly Journal of Medicine,* **28,** 235–258.
British Medical Journal (1974) Leading article. The assessment and management of acromegaly. *British Medical Journal,* 549–550.
Evered, D. C. (1974) Diseases of the thyroid. *Clinics in Endocrinology and Metabolism,* **3,** 425–450.
Forsyth, I. & Edwards, C. R.W. (1972) Human prolactin, its isolation, assay and clinical applications. *Clinical Endocrinology,* **1,** 293–314.
Greenwood, F. C., Landon, J. & Stamp, T. C. B. (1966) The plasma sugar, free fatty acid, cortisol and growth hormone response to insulin. *Journal of Clinical Investigation,* **45,** 429–436.
Hall, R. (1972) The immunoassay of thyroid-stimulating hormone and its clinical applications. *Clinical Endocrinology,* **1,** 115–125.
Hall, R. (1973) The hypothalamic control of the pituitary. *British Journal of Hospital Medicine,* **9,** 109–113.
Hall, R., Evered, D. C. & Tunbridge, W. M. G. (1973) The role of thyroid stimulating hormone and thyrotrophin-releasing hormone in thyroid disease. *9th Symposium on Advanced Medicine.* pp.15–26. London: Pitman Medical.

Hall, R., Anderson, J., Smart, G. A. & Besser, G. M. (1974) *Fundamentals of Clinical Endocrinology*, 2nd edition. London: Pitman Medical.

Hoffenberg, R. (1974) Aetiology of hyperthyroidism. *British Medical Journal*, iii, 452–456.

Lancet (1974) Leading article. Growth-hormone release-inhibiting hormone . *Lancet*, i, 1148–1150.

Mattingly, D. & Tyler, C. (1967) Simple screening test for Cushing's syndrome. *British Medical Journal*, iv, 394–397.

Mortimer, C., Besser, G. M., McNeilly, A. S., Marshall, J. C., Harsoulis, P., Tunbridge, W. M. G., Gomez-Pan, A. & Hall, R. (1973) Luteinising hormone and follicle stimulating hormone-releasing hormone test in patients with hypothalamic-pituitary-gonadal dysfunction. *British Medical Journal*, iv, 73–77.

Newton, J. R., Ramsay, I. & Marsden, P. (1971) Clomiphene as a test of pituitary function. *Lancet*, ii, 190–192.

Pittman, J. A. (1974) Thyrotrophin-releasing hormone. *Advances in Internal Medicine*, 19, 303–325.

Raiti, S. & Maclaren, N. K. (1974) Advances in human growth hormone research. *Federation Proceedings*, 33, 1682–1685.

Short, R. V. (1972) The control of menstruation. *British Journal of Hospital Medicine*, 7, 552–555.

CHAPTER FOUR

Ophthalmological Aspects of Pituitary Tumours

A. L. CROMBIE

The chiasmal area is of great importance to ophthalmologists, not only because lesions in this area often cause ophthalmic symptoms and signs but also because these ophthalmological manifestations may be the only presenting ones. An 'awareness' on the part of the ophthalmologist is therefore essential if delays in diagnosis are not to occur. Delays do, however, occur and this chapter is written in the hope that it may help to alert clinicians to the many ways in which pituitary lesions present and to some practical ways of facilitating what can be a very difficult clinical diagnosis. The general signs and symptoms of pituitary tumours have been dealt with elsewhere; hence the purely ophthalmological slant to this section which is based on a personal series of 100 patients with chromophobe adenoma of the pituitary, 150 cases of acromegaly, 30 cases of Cushing's syndrome, 20 cases of craniopharyngioma and 20 heterogenous types of chiasmal lesions.

ANATOMICAL CONSIDERATIONS

The key to the relationship between field defects and tumours in the region of the optic chiasm is the anatomy of the chiasm in which 60 per cent of nerve fibres in the chiasm decussate in alternate laminae and cross. Some of these anterior decussating fibres form a short loop extruding into the optic nerve of the opposite side before passing posteriorly to the optic tract of that side, while more posterior fibres do the same vis-à-vis the homolateral optic tract before crossing. These loops give rise to atypical field defects but can be of great localising value. Macular fibres decussate in the same manner as peripheral fibres but do so in the posterior portion of the chiasm and lesions impinging on this region give rise to central scotomatous defects. There are, no doubt, individual variations in the precise location and numbers of crossing fibres in any chiasm and these variations can give rise to diagnostic confusion. There is also a considerable variation in the anatomical relationship between the sella turcica and the chiasm which is of importance in the development of field defects. In the majority of people (79 per cent) the posterior border of the chiasm lies directly over the dorsum sellae, while in another five per cent the chiasm lies partially on the tuberculum. In a very few people (one to two per cent) the chiasm lies behind the dorsum sellae and in the remaining 12 per cent of people the chiasm lies on the diaphragm (Schaeffer, 1924). This variation of chiasmal position, the pre- and post-fixed chiasm, coupled with variations of blood supply and crossing of fibres in the chiasm, is the reason why the classical bitemporal field defect of chiasmal disease in which the chiasm is completely transected is rarer than was first thought. A recent study emphasises that the decussation of fibres in the optic chiasm is supplied primarily by inferiorly located blood vessels (Bergland and Ray, 1969) and this no doubt is of great significance in the production of chiasmal field defects, but it must be remembered that the chiasmal blood supply is provided by a plexus of arterial branches derived from the surrounding intracranial vessels which include the anterior cerebral, the internal carotid, the anterior and posterior communicating arteries and the hypophyseal artery.

In the chiasmal syndrome much interest has centred on the preservation of the upper nasal field. In a study of fresh postmortem material Hedges (1969) has shown that during expansion of an intrasellar mass the upper temporal fibres coursing in the lateral aspect of the chiasm increase in axial length while the lower temporal fibres (the upper nasal quadrant) decrease in axial length. This probable relaxation sustains the blood supply for longer than other parts of the chiasm not so relaxed, hence the preservation of the upper nasal quadrant of field. The last anatomical point of note is that the chiasm lies well above the diaphragma sellae and that considerable expansion of a pituitary adenoma – at least 5 to 10 mm – upwards has to take place before the chiasm is involved.

ADVANCES IN OPHTHALMOLOGICAL EXAMINATION TECHNIQUES

Examination of visual fields

During recent years a number of hemispherical perimeters with projected light stimuli have been developed. The advantage of these perimeters over the Bjerrum screen and the arc perimeters are (1) that the background illumination is standardised, the stimulus being altered in size and intensity and (2) that fixation can be monitored. The two main types of hemispherical projection perimeters are the Goldmann perimeter (Goldmann, 1945), and the Tubingen (Oculus) perimeter (Harms, 1950). Both these perimeters have a short working distance, the consequence of which is that the central 30° field is portrayed and tested over a small area, although the Tubingen perimeter is better in this respect than the Goldmann perimeter. In the author's view, since the central fields are vital in chiasmal disease, projection perimeters are no substitute for a careful examination of the visual fields on a 2 m Bjerrum screen where subtleties of field change in this area can be magnified and analysed comprehensively. Until recently nearly all testing of visual fields was done using kinetic perimetry, plotting many isopters with different stimuli. This allowed an estimate of the slope of the defect.

A newer technique of perimetry, static perimetry, has found favour of late. This technique produces a map of the visual fields by uncovering the differential threshold of many points in the visual field, using stationary stimuli, and then joining all those points in the visual field which have the same threshold. The field is not recorded in isopters but along meridians. The advocates of static perimetry feel that central scotomas are well analysed by this method. The method is, however, time-consuming and needs a great deal of patient cooperation. In spite of the claims of static perimetrists the author feels that in chiasmal disease the use of the Bjerrum screen is mandatory and that one of the most subtle ways of eliciting field defects on a Bjerrum screen is by reducing the illumination, a technique which should be used more often by clinical neuro-ophthalmologists. In the author's series no field defect was missed on a Bjerrum screen examination using this technique that was later picked up on a projection perimeter. Another way of reducing the stimulus is by the use of coloured test objects, in particular a 5-mm red object in chiasmal disease. This technique as well as reductions in illumination will elicit the earliest and most subtle of field changes.

Apparent visual field defects

In the examination of visual fields great care must be taken to eliminate possible sources of error since this examination is, despite more sophisticated means of testing, in the final analysis, subjective. It is because of this that the author firmly believes that the testing of visual fields should be carried out only after a thorough ophthalmological examination and preferably the field tester should be the ophthalmologist himself.

Physical causes of apparent visual field defects

Refractive errors

In perimetry in which a working distance of 330 cm is used the correction of refractive errors is extremely significant because fixation is so critical at this short working distance. Not only can refractive errors, especially myopia, appear to produce field defects but if a true field defect is present this may be exaggerated or changed to a degree in which accurate localisation of the causative lesion is made much more difficult. In uncorrected aphakia the visual field appears contracted because of poor visual acuity and if such a patient is being tested large fixation objects will have to be used. The corrected aphakic patient also presents a problem in relation to perimetry in so far as the inherent spherical aberration of an aphakic correction prevents the examination of the visual fields outside the central 25° as well as causing a 'roving scotoma' to appear. The wearing of contact lenses by an aphakic patient improves the quality of perimetry but the visual field is still reduced by 25° to 30° compared to normal at the periphery of the field.

Anomalies of lid and brow

In acromegaly where there is marked overgrowth of the orbital ridges, apparent bitemporal defects can be produced. The same type of defects can also appear as the result of ptosis of the upper lid from whatever cause, while in elderly patients blepharochalasis may often produce bitemporal field defects unless the loose skin is taped up to the forehead.

Corneal and Lens Opacities

Any appreciable corneal or lens opacity may cause a generalised contraction of field and may well accentuate any field defect. Corneal opacities usually cause a field defect on the side of the lesion while opacities in the lens, particularly in the posterior cortical region, may well have the opposite effect.

Enlargement of the blind spot associated with optic nerve head anomalies and pathology

If enlargement of the blind spot is found on perimetry great care should be taken in its evaluation since the enlargement may well be due to intrinsic changes at the nerve head of no neuro-ophthalmological significance. Such intrinsic changes can be divided into two groups, congenital and acquired. The congenital anomalies include drusen body formation at the disc, myelination of retinal nerve fibres at the nerve head, colobomas of the disc including inferior conus, and myopia. The acquired changes at the disc include true papilloedema, juxtapapillary choroiditis, peripapillary choroidal atrophy and disc changes resulting from open-angle glaucoma.

Other causes of apparent visual field defects

A patient who is ill may well find cooperation difficult and in these circumstances speed of testing is essential so that the best use can be made of the patient's faculties. Apart from the difficulties of fixation another common difficulty is slowness of response and a dulling of perceptual awareness in relation to test objects. When this occurs it may well be necessary to move objects from seeing to blind areas rather than the normal opposite procedure; this causes the field to be approximately 5° different from normal. Malingering and hysteria produce problems in perimetry but the hallmark of malingering is the field which stays the same size irrespective of size of object while the hallmark of the hysteric is the field which spirals down to fixation using the same object size.

Fluorescence Angiography

In 1960, Novotny and Alvis introduced the techniques of fluorescence angiography or fluorography as it is now called. This technique is of great use in relation to chiasmal syndromes where there is doubt as to whether or not the optic disc is swollen or atrophic. Fluorography can demonstrate the capillary network on the disc head with ease and the state of this network can give vital information regarding pathology in this region. If the network is increased and extra capillaries are seen and, in the later phases, some extravascular leakage of fluorescein is seen, papilloedema can be diagnosed even in its very early stages. If, on the other hand, there is a dearth of capillaries on the nerve head and there is doubtful pallor of the disc, optic atrophy can be diagnosed with confidence. Confusion has reigned in the literature regarding the nomenclature of optic atrophy. The author subscribes to the view that optic atrophy is only present if there is a demonstrable loss of optic nerve function and, if there is no such loss of function, pallor of the optic disc is the term which should be used.

Red free light

The use of red free light in fundal examination has been well documented (Hoyt, Sehlicke and Eckethoff, 1972) but recently attention has been focussed on this simple examination method again in relation to the nerve fibre layer of the retina. Using a suitable filter in an ophthalmoscope the nerve fibre layer can be clearly seen, as can gaps in it, which are of great importance when they occur in the areas adjacent to the disc and where optic atrophy and field defects have been found.

Optic Nerve Conduction Studies

Reference will be made to the difficulties experienced in the diagnosis of optic atrophy in patients with chiasmal disease. The techniques of electro-encephalography as applied to the VER and computerisation have made possible objective measurements on the state of optic nerve conduction in optic neuritis (Halliday et al, 1972). It is the author's firm belief that this technique will be of value in patients with chiasmal disease where the state of the optic nerve is difficult to ascertain by clinical methods. The technique of eliciting the visual evoked response (VER) is painless and non-invasive and would seem to be worthy of trial in chiasmal disease as a useful adjunct to clinical examination, particularly since the use of a patterned stimulus has improved the effectiveness of the VER because of the greater neuronal area which such a pattern stimulates with a simple flash stimulus.

OCULAR SYMPTOMS

The ocular symptoms of chiasmal and parachiasmal lesions are chiefly related to visual field defects and defective visual acuity. The classical field defect in chiasmal lesions is bitemporal hemianopia which the patient may well ignore until the degree of field loss is gross. If the bitemporal field loss is total, two other visual symptoms may appear upon which little emphasis has been placed by clinicians up to the present. The first is the chiasmatic post-fixational blindness syndrome (Blakemore, 1970), in which a patient who develops a complete bitemporal hemianopia no longer has any areas in his remaining hemiretinas which have corresponding visual points and is therefore incapable of binocular single vision. An object just beyond the point of fixation will disappear as it is in both temporal fields while an object closer than fixation will result in disparate images in the two visual fields which will not disappear. Such a patient will learn that if he sees two disparate images they come from an object closer than fixation, and that he has a scotoma just beyond the object of fixation. The second phenomenon resulting from a complete bitemporal hemianopia is that a type of diplopia, the hemifield slide phenomenon (Kirkham, 1972) can occur because of the lack of binocular single vision. If the patient's eyes remain straight, the two remaining half fields will touch along the central vertical meridian but, if the eyes diverge, the two half fields will overlap and diplopia will result, in the absence of extra-ocular muscle paralysis. Conversely, if the patient's eyes converge, he will have to develop alternation of fixation, otherwise objects will disappear just temporal to fixation. If the patient has a vertical heterotropia he may complain of vertical steps in the horizon which can cause marked confusion since space orientation often hinges on an unbroken horizon. The classical example of the hemifield slide phenomenon occurring vertically is the patient who sees a lake at two levels without a waterfall. The hemifield slide phenomenon has in the past accounted for a number of reports of diplopia in chiasmal lesions which have exaggerated the true incidence of nerve palsies in these conditions. The true incidence of extra-ocular muscle palsies in chiasmal disease is difficult to quantify but in the author's experience the incidence in intrasellar tumours is four per cent. Diplopia due to extra-ocular muscle palsies in suprasellar and parasellar lesions is much higher and is in the region of 20 per cent, and when pain is also present, is indicative of parasellar disease.

While patients are aware of diplopia, loss of visual acuity in one eye is often overlooked for a long time and becomes apparent only when the good eye is covered for one reason or another. Knight, Hoyt and Wilson (1972) have drawn attention to the visual disturbance produced by pressure on an optic nerve in front of the chiasm by a meningioma or a pituitary adenoma. This visual disturbance takes the form of a vague but persistent dimming of vision in which loss of visual acutity is not measurable, and there is no disc pallor. There is an apparent pupillary defect however and colour vision is impaired. Loss of visual acuity is an important symptom in chiasmal lesions since a number of these lesions present with central scotomas. Such a scotoma, if hemianopic, characterises the lesion as chiasmal and not due to lesions in the optic tract or geniculo-calcarine pathway where visual acuity is not impaired unless the lesion is bilateral.

Headache

Headache is a common feature of pituitary disease. In the author's series the incidence of headache was greatest amongst patients with acromegaly, being 55 per cent. The incidence in patients with chromophobe adenoma was 40 per cent. The headaches are often difficult to localise, but if they can be, the supra-orbital region seems to be the most common site followed by pain either in or around the eyes. In a few cases sensitivity to light is an added feature of the headaches which can occasionally lead to a misdiagnosis of migraine. Classically, headaches worsen when an intrasellar tumour is pressing on the diaphragma sellae and then become much less after an acute exacerbation during which the tumour has burst through the diaphragma sellae. In the author's experience this classical history is rare and he has never seen pituitary headache worsened by the ingestion of sugar as described by Pardee (1919).

Ocular signs of pituitary tumour

Reference has already been made to diplopia and extra-ocular muscle palsies and to loss of visual acuity in the section on symptoms, and it is not proposed to deal with them any further.

Optic Atrophy and Pallor of the optic disc

Optic atrophy has been described in more than half the patients harbouring pituitary tumours. The diagnosis of optic atrophy has been based upon degree of pallor of the disc as observed by the clinician or by photography. Visual function in many cases of so-called optic atrophy is good and the opposite is also true. Thus in the author's opinion, optic atrophy should describe pallor of the disc associated with defective vision and/or visual field defects, while a pale disc with associated good vision and no visual field defects should be described simply as showing pallor. This distinction is not just a question of semantics but serves to distinguish pathological processes. A pale disc with good visual function, etc is probably the seat of reactive glial overgrowth and a degree of fibrosis as well as a loss of superficial capillaries on the disc surface. A pale disc associated with poor visual function is the seat of true axonal degeneration since the optic nerve fibres are the axons of the retinal ganglion cells and optic atrophy is the final common manifestation of lesions of either one or the other. A sign which may be of help in trying to diagnose pallor or optic atrophy, as compared to the normal variations in colour of the disc, is a reduction of the number of arterioles on the disc from an average of 10 to less than seven. Little help is given by the calibre of the retinal vessels as these are often within normal limits in most cases of optic atrophy or pallor of the disc. The optic discs may appear pale and yet be atrophic in a number of ophthalmological conditions, the commonest being myopia, varying types of congenital colobomas and senile peripapillary changes. It is therefore vital that before optic atrophy is diagnosed and extensive investigations undertaken a thorough and competent ophthalmological examination is carried out. In a very small number of pituitary tumours, but in approximately 15 per cent of suprasellar tumours, papilloedema may ensue which can be followed by secondary optic atrophy. Once this has happened further papilloedema will be unlikely and this important diagnostic sign may be lost.

The use of fluorescein angiography has helped greatly to elucidate nerve head circulatory changes and hence the diagnosis of optic atrophy. In cases of pituitary tumour, if there is minimal optic atrophy of short duration, some return to normality at the disc head may occur but if the optic atrophy is of long standing and vision has been defective for some time no such return can be expected.

Pupillary signs

Pupillomotor signs can be of great clinical help in the diagnosis of optic nerve conduction defects and in cases of pituitary tumour they are almost wholly correlative. It is very rare for intrasellar tumours, while remaining in the sella, to produce pupillary signs although parasellar lesions, particularly aneurysms, often do so. Clinically therefore it can occasionally be a problem to decide whether pupillary involvement is the result of optic nerve damage or separate oculomotor nerve dysfunction. A full examination will usually sort this out but the author has seen cases where only extensive investigation has produced the answer.

Visual Field Defects

Visual field defects in chiasmal lesions are probably the most helpful signs in the localisation of such disease and it is the author's belief that these field defects can be best demonstrated on the 2 m Bjerrum screen. There are four main groups of lesions which will cause pressure on the chiasm and in all of these the early field defects are demonstrable on the Bjerrum screen provided the perimetrist has screen lighting which can be varied and, in particular, can be reduced in intensity. Pressure on the chiasm can arise in the midline from below, e.g. a chromophobe adenoma, or from above, e.g. a craniopharyngioma or aneurysm, in which case the field defects may be classically bitemporal and hemianopic in type, the only difference being in which temporal quadrants the field defects first appear. Pressure on the antero-lateral angle of the chiasm, e.g. a chromophobe adenoma or an inner sphenoidal ridge meningioma, will cause initially a central scotoma on the side of the lesion with a peripheral temporal defect in the other eye. Lastly, pressure on the postero-lateral angle of the chiasm will produce not only a chiasmal defect but also a homonymous hemianopic defect, as the optic tract may well be involved. It is worthy of note that the third ventricle is capable of distension in internal hydrocephalus to such a degree that it can act as an extrasellar 'tumour' and cause bitemporal hemianopia. Wagener and Cusick (1937) were of the opinion that the usual underlying cause for third ventricular dilatation of this magnitude was a tumour in the posterior fossa, but it is probably more frequently a consequence of longstanding congenital stenosis of the aqueduct. Binasal hemianopia is exceedingly rare and is reportedly due to a displacement of the third ventricle which in turn displaces the chiasm anteriorly so that the internal carotid arteries cause compression of the uncrossed fibres from the temporal halves of the retinae.

In the author's experience the majority of cases of pituitary tumours had bitemporal defects which behaved in the classical manner as regards progression. However, a much smaller number of cases had bitemporal, hemianopic central defects with or without peripheral defects. Purely unilateral, central scotomas were also seen as well as total blindness in one eye and temporal hemianopia in the other. The variety of visual field defects in chiasmal disease would seem to emphasise that the visual field presentation in such cases is infinitely variable and that central as well as peripheral defects must be looked for. Another important point regarding those visual field defects described above is that asymmetry is as common as symmetry and this can on occasions be misleading in terms of an early definitive diagnosis of chiasmal disease. Unilateral arcuate field defects have been described in pituitary tumours (Kearns and Rucker, 1957) due to initial optic nerve involvement on one side only, but the author has never seen such a case.

Nystagmus

An unusual type of nystagmus has been described in cases of chromophobe adenoma of the pituitary, called see-saw nystagmus. It is a pendular, dissociated nystagmus with the eyes rising and falling alternately and with associated torsional nystagmus. The characteristics occur at a higher amplitude and lower frequency on downward gaze. Fein and Williams (1969) reviewed the literature and found 15 cases in the world, ten of these cases being associated with sellar and parasellar disease. The remaining five cases suffered from miscellaneous forms of brain stem disease. The author has seen two cases of see-saw nystagmus, one occurring in a patient with a large chromophobe adenoma and the other in a patient with vascular brain stem disease. The mechanisms responsible for see-saw nystagmus are probably represented on multiple levels and the entity should not be equated specifically with other signs traditionally associated with parasellar disease. See-saw nystagmus has been reported as occurring after traumatic bitemporal hemianopia (Fisher et al, 1968) and Maddox (1913) asserted that bitemporal hemianopia was a prerequisite for the development of this rare sign. The author has seen no other cases of nystagmus in his series of chiasmal pathology but monocular nystagmus has been described in two cases at eight months and three years, in which this sign was the first indication of the chiasmal tumours affecting these children (Donin, 1967).

PITUITARY ADENOMA

Chromophobe Adenoma

As stated earlier the author's series consists of 100 cases, 55 males and 45 females, and the age incidence is shown in Table 4.1. Reference has already been made to the incidence of extra-ocular muscle palsies in this series being four per cent though diplopia was complained of in 20 per cent.

Table 4.1. Age incidence of chromophobe adenoma 100 cases studied.

Age (years)	Per cent of cases
Under 20	2
20–29	10
30–39	17
40–49	34
50–59	25
60–69	12

There has been much controversy in the literature regarding the incidence and type of field defects in chromophobe adenoma, Lyle and Clover (1961) citing an incidence of bitemporal hemianopic field defects of 79 per cent while Wilson and Falconer (1968) put this defect as low as 36 per cent in their series. In addition, Wilson and Falconer remarked on the high incidence of bitemporal hemianopic scotomatous defects – 48 per cent in their series, which they felt was a defect to which insufficient attention had been paid. In the author's series, 65 per cent of cases had bitemporal hemianopic field defects with no scotomatous defects when first examined. However, a further 21 per cent had bitemporal hemianopic scotomas, as described above, but in about half of these cases *peripheral temporal hemianopic field defects were present as well*. Five cases (five per cent) had homonymous hemianopic field defects, while four per cent had *unilateral central scotomas with no defect in the other eye*. A further five cases had unilateral central scotomas with a temporal peripheral field defect in the other eye and the remaining five cases were blind in one eye with a temporal hemianopia in the other. This variation of field defect in chromophobe adenoma has been highlighted by others (Elkington, 1968) and emphasises the necessity for a high degree of awareness of such variability on the part of the ophthalmologist or neurologist. Jefferson (1940), in a classical paper on extrasellar expansion of pituitary tumours, pointed out how such variability could occur. This multiplicity of routes for expansion, coupled with the anatomical variables already alluded to, can cause the utmost confusion in the diagnosis of chromophobe adenomas. All the patients in the present series had field defects, but only 56 (56 per cent) had definite optic atrophy. This fact has often been emphasised and this series only serves to emphasise the point that definite and dense visual field defects as well as lowered visual acuity can occur in the presence of what seems to be a normal optic nerve head. It may well be, however, that optic nerve conduction studies will show that there is pathological optic nerve conduction in the presence of normal gross anatomy of the nerve. Conversely, some patients with what seemed to be dense optic atrophy had minimal peripheral field defects. This variability of association of visible optic nerve changes and visual field defects is one of the factors which can be misleading in chiasmal disease and is a contributory cause to the often delayed diagnosis in these cases. In the present series there is, on average, an interval of at least two years between the onset of symptoms and a definitive diagnosis being made and verified. The behaviour of the field defects in the cases reviewed has followed along classical lines in that the bitemporal hemianopic defects, often asymmetric, have progressed slowly and have stopped at the vertical meridian. The field defects seem to equalise in this position and after an interval may progress again. The character of the edge of the defect has also been of help in indicating the possible speed of progression of the defects – a shallow edge indicating a faster rate of expansion than a steep edge. The scotomatous defects seemed to progress at a faster rate than the non-scotomatous defects and this is in agreement with Wilson and Falconer (1968). An important point is that if such central defects do progress rapidly central vision will be lost at a much earlier stage than if a peripheral visual field defect had been present. Visual loss of this kind will, of course, bring the patient to see a doctor more quickly than if a peripheral field defect had been present. This in turn is probably responsible for the extremely good visual results in patients with scotomatous defects. Following treatment, all the scotomatous field defects regressed or disappeared. The peripheral field defects recovered fully in 25 per cent of cases, 45 per cent improved greatly, 25 per cent improved partially and 5 per cent became worse. This last group in the main harboured large tumours which had been present for a long time and had caused considerable surgical difficulty.

It is also of note that in this series of chromophobe adenomas not one case of papilloedema was seen. Elkington (1968) saw papilloedema in only one case out of 260 and this seems to be the general experience. If a normal optic nerve head is present, even though visual field defects are present, a good visual prognosis is indicated in the author's experience, provided the surgery, etc. is uncomplicated. It is worth emphasising that in five patients in the series complete blindness was present in one eye with a dense temporal hemianopia in the other. The author has seen a case identical in clinical findings which was finally diagnosed and proved to be an anterior communicating aneurysm (Cullen, Haining and Crombie, 1966) so that angiography is obviously a necessity in the investigation of chiasmal lesions.

ACROMEGALY

The author has examined an unusually large number of patients suffering from acromegaly, 150 in all. An equal sex incidence, a peak age incidence of 35 to 40 years, a history of headache in 50 per cent of the cases and an average interval of approximately three to five years between onset of symptoms and diagnosis make this series a fairly standard one when compared to others in the literature. All the patients had enlargement of the sella turcica on detailed x-ray measurement and, of those who had air encephalography, only one per cent showed suprasellar extension of any kind. Growth hormone levels were measured and found to be raised in all the pretreatment cases. Lillie (1925) described a series of 50 patients with acromegaly and found field defects in 32 per cent. This is not the author's experience and in this series of 150 patients only three patients had chiasmal field defects prior to treatment and only one case had optic atrophy, this last case having had surgery for an eosinophil adenoma in another centre. No cases of extra-ocular muscle palsies have been noted, nor of proptosis. In short, from the ophthalmological point of view, acromegaly seems to constitute an extremely limited threat to the visual apparatus as evidenced by this series. In Newcastle upon Tyne the therapeutic approach to acromegaly has been an active one in the hope of improving the poor cardiovascular prognosis in these cases. The main therapeutic weapon has been transphenoidal implantation of ^{90}yttrium seeds into the pituitary gland. This carries a minor surgical risk which is discussed elsewhere but the ocular complications are not negligible. An incidence of 10 per cent of extra-ocular muscle palsies has been noted following treatment, the third cranial nerve being most affected in 80 per cent of cases and the sixth cranial nerve accounting for the remainder. These palsies have been transient, coming on usually within three to four days of implantation and lasting for up to six weeks. Field defects have also been noted in this series, occurring in five per cent of cases so treated and usually taking the form of unilateral temporal field loss or unilateral temporal, central scotomatous defects. In all the cases save two these field defects have been transitory and are no doubt due to a direct radiation effect, oedema or a vascular effect at the junction of the optic nerve and chiasm. In two cases the field defects were permanent and unilateral optic atrophy ensued. With the advent of growth hormone blocking agents such as CB 134, the need for radiation in case of acromegaly may well decline if such drugs fulfil their early promise. The only case of pituitary apoplexy in the whole of the author's series of pituitary tumours occurred in an acromegalic patient who had severe acromegaly which had been surgically treated elsewhere. This treatment had been followed by external irradiation on two occasions because of continuing symptoms and raised growth hormone levels. While in hospital for further investigation he developed sudden unilateral proptosis with severe pain and total ophthalmoplegia and died within two hours of the onset of these signs. Pituitary apoplexy is said to be more common in acromegaly than in other pituitary tumours (Brougham, Heusner and Adams, 1950) and at times has resulted from x-ray therapy to the tumour (Crompton and Layton, 1961). Prompt neurosurgery can be beneficial in cases of pituitary apoplexy but in the case described above was not considered because of his poor general condition. No preceding history of sneezing or coughing occurred in this patient, although this has been incriminated in some cases as a cause of haemorrhage into a pituitary tumour due to raised venous pressure in the cavernous sinus (Dawson and Kothandaram, 1972).

CUSHING'S SYNDROME

The author has seen 20 cases of Cushing's syndrome and none of them was thought to be primarily of pituitary origin. Rovit and Berry (1965) and Salassa et al (1959), however, have assessed a total of 67 cases of Cushing's syndrome resulting from a pituitary tumour, only 10 per cent of cases of the syndrome originating in this way. From the series mentioned above a number of points of interest can be noted.

1. The pituitary tumours in Cushing's syndrome seem to be active and relatively fast growing.
2. Twenty-five per cent of patients with Cushing's syndrome and pituitary tumours have extra-ocular muscle palsies, an incidence two to four times that of the same palsies in non-secreting chromophobe adenomas. The third nerve is most frequently affected.
3. Adrenalectomy may incite the development of a pituitary tumour in Cushing's syndrome and this may result in hyperpigmentation.

The author has seen three such cases of Nelson's syndrome (Nelson et al, 1958) in whom no overt neuro-ophthalmological signs were present despite the marked pigmentation. The literature suggests that pituitary tumours induced by adrenalectomy expand rapidly and are composed of ACTH secreting cells rather than of basophilic cells.

4. The field defects in the pituitary tumours of Cushing's syndrome are rarely of the classical bitemporal type but often produce scotomatous types of defect and, in a significant number, a homonymous type of defect, i.e. optic tract involvement $\pm$ chiasmal involvement. These tumours, therefore, though rare, do seem to differ from the classical chromophobe types in their behaviour as regards growth, types of field defect and incidence of extra-ocular muscle palsies.

CRANIOPHARYNGIOMAS

While craniopharyngiomas are classically described as occurring mainly in the first two decades of life, in the author's series, another significant group manifests itself in the fifth decade. Histologically, the craniopharyngiomas in these two age groups have been identical, but the stimulus that leads to probable bursts of growth remains unknown. Forty per cent of craniopharyngiomas occurred in the fifth decade or later in the author's series and this is in accord with some other series (Wise et al, 1955). In the present series sudden onset of symptoms or acute exacerbations of symptoms have not been seen as described by Bhagwati and Vuckovich (1963) and ascribed to either rupture of the cysts or inundation of the adjacent structures and cerebrospinal fluid by irritative cyst contents, all the patients having had symptoms attributable to a slow-growing, space-occupying lesion in the region of the chiasm. In the series 95 per cent of patients complained of headache and 70 per cent of vomiting suggestive of at least intermittently raised intracranial pressure. Visual loss, either of acuity or visual field or both, occurred in 80 per cent of the cases; and optic disc changes, either of papilloedema or optic atrophy or of papilloedema superimposed on optic atrophy, occurred in all the cases. This last combination seems to be of great importance in the younger group of patients with craniopharyngiomas, as the centre of the disc remains pale and the oedema occurs at the periphery giving it the appearance of cupping, such as that found in open-angle glaucoma. Matson and Crigler (1969) described a series of 57 cases of childhood craniopharyngioma in whom visual field defects were found in 33 cases (58%) and papilloedema in 30 (53%) cases. In the present series visual field changes occurred in 80 per cent of the cases, papilloedema occurred in 20 per cent, papilloedema and optic atrophy in 10 per cent and optic atrophy or pallor in 70 per cent. The visual field defects, often difficult to chart properly in the youngest children, were in general asymmetrical which is in agreement with Wagener and Love (1943), probably reflecting the asymmetrical growth of these embryonal cysts. The classical picture of bitemporal hemianopia with the lower temporal quadrants affected first occurred in only four cases of the twenty; in a further four cases blindness in one eye and a temporal field defect in the other were found. There were central and paracentral scotomas in six cases and in the remaining six cases with field defects an optic tract type of hemianopia was found – no doubt reflecting the posterior position of some craniopharyngiomas compared to tumours of pituitary origin. The degree of optic atrophy was at times difficult to correlate with the degree of field loss and it is well known that optic atrophy usually lags behind loss of vision by varying degrees in any one patient. The high incidence of visual field changes and optic nerve changes no doubt reflects the ophthalmological character of the series. In patients with papilloedema only, and these were nearly all in the younger age group, the signs of increased intracranial pressure predominated. These included sixth nerve palsies in four of the six cases with papilloedema. The diplopia and sixth nerve palsies cleared rapidly after the increased intracranial pressure had been reduced by surgical means. On the other hand no field defect completely disappeared following neurosurgery, which is in accord with the findings of others (Campbell and Ball, 1972). If surgery resulted in incomplete removal of the cyst recurrence of ocular symptoms and signs occurred in 30 per cent within two years. Complete removal of the cyst produced the best visual results with no recurrences. One case of interest concerned a boy aged 19 with a craniopharyngioma, bilateral optic atrophy and bitemporal field defects. A radical excision of the cyst was not possible and because of recurrences radioactive colloidal ^{90}yttrium was injected into the cyst in an effort to kill off the living epithelial secreting cells. Bilateral lower altitudinal field defects followed this procedure which are total and static. The colloidal ^{90}yttrium sedimented to the lowest part of the cyst which overlies the chiasm and the author's surmise is that the altitudinal field defects are due to chiasmal damage from radiation by the colloidal ^{90}yttrium.

MENINGIOMAS

The chiasmal syndrome can be produced by olfactory groove and sphenoidal ridge meningiomas but the group which characteristically produces the chiasmal syndrome is composed of those arising from the tuberculum sellae. In contrast to suprasellar meningiomas, olfactory groove and sphenoidal ridge meningiomas produce chiasmal signs when the tumours have attained a considerable size. Posterior extension of posteriorly rising olfactory groove meningioma involves the chiasm, the sella turcica and the hypophyseal stalk. Hartmann, David and Dasirgues (1937) found that papilloedema occurred in 56 per cent of their cases while Huber (1961) observed a Foster–Kennedy syndrome in 15 per cent of his cases. The author has seen three cases of olfactory groove meningiomas responsible for a chiasmal syndrome. All three cases had papilloedema more pronounced on one side than the other but this finding was of no use in lateralising the tumour, and ocular movements and pupil reactions were normal. All three cases had paracentral scotomas with bilateral peripheral hemianopic field defects which regressed completely following successful surgery, although the optic nerve heads became slightly pale. Meningiomas of the inner third of the sphenoidal ridge are those which may rarely produce a chiasmal syndrome. Classically these tumours produce cranial nerve palsies, the sixth nerve being most commonly involved, exophthalmos of varying degree and optic atrophy on the side involved followed by papilloedema on the other side. In the author's series four cases of inner third sphenoidal ridge meningiomas produced chiasmal signs. All these cases had optic atrophy on the affected side by the time they were seen, associated with early papilloedema in the contralateral eye in two cases and optic atrophy only in the remaining two cases. Visual loss was marked on the affected side and the field defects involved central and paracentral scotomas and early temporal field defects on the unaffected side. The field defects on the unaffected side reduced following surgery but in two of the four cases central scotomas and visual loss persisted. One of the cases had a partial third nerve palsy prior to surgery which resolved subsequently and two of the cases had mild exophthalmos prior to surgery. As has been pointed out, suprasellar meningiomas are by far the commonest of the meningiomas to cause chiasmal signs and symptoms. The usual age of occurrence is between the ages of 30 and 50 and both sexes are affected equally. Cushing (1930) in a classical paper described the suprasellar meningioma as causing 'primary optic atrophy with bitemporal field defects in an adult patient showing an essentially normal sella turcica.' In the main these are slow-growing tumours, often discovered late and malignant change is rare, but if the tumour arises in a child scotomatous change is not uncommon (Russel and Rubinstein, 1963). The author has not examined any children with suprasellar meningiomas but has seen nine adult cases, four females and five males with an average age of 48 years. Six of the cases had bilateral optic atrophy, more marked in one eye than the other in three of them, while one patient had unilateral optic atrophy and a normal fundus in the other eye. The two remaining cases had normal fundi but one had a partial third nerve palsy – the only patient in the series to have an extra-ocular muscle palsy – while the other patient showed classical bitemporal field defects. This last finding emphasises an ill-reported point concerning suprasellar meningiomas and that is that field defects often bear little relation to the fundal findings. The field defects are, as a rule, very asymmetrical and this may be helpful in the differential diagnosis. Three other patients had bitemporal field defects which were much more advanced in one eye than the other. Three patients had unilateral central scotomatous defects, presumably due to prechiasmic region involvement, with early temporal field defects in the other eye, and one patient had a paracentral hemianopic defect due to involvement of the postchiasmal region. The remaining patient, with the third nerve palsy had no field defects whatsoever on the most detailed testing. Any correlation between the degree of optic atrophy and the extent and density of the field defects was difficult to attain. It is stated that suprasellar meningiomas account for a higher proportion of patients with papilloedema (Walsh and Hoyt, 1969) but in the author's limited experience this is not so. Following surgery the above nine cases all showed a significant reduction in the field defects but no changes in the atrophic discs. The single third nerve palsy resolved completely. In all the above cases the tumours were moderately large but earlier diagnosis would no doubt have made surgery easier and in this respect a high index of suspicion and angiography are of the greatest importance.

OTHER TUMOURS

A number of rarer tumours occur in the chiasmal region and the following section deals with such tumours as have occurred in the author's series.

Chiasmal glioma

Chiasmal glioma usually occurs in association with optic nerve gliomas or with those of the third ventricle and frontal lobe which extend through the leptomeninges. There are, however, a few cases of intrinsic glioma of the chiasm and the author has examined one such case which was diagnosed on physical findings, air encephalography and its course over a number of years. The case in question is a female aged 24 with familial neurofibromatosis, static bitemporal defects with optic atrophy and a thickened chiasm. No treatment has been given and the field defects have remained static for five years.

Glaser, Hoyt and Corbett (1971) reported on the long-term prognosis of such cases and felt that irradiation was of no value and that the long-term visual prognosis was good, which would seem to be in agreement with the author's very limited experience.

Chordoma

The author has seen one case of a chordoma causing a chiasmal syndrome in a 45-year-old female. As well as optic atrophy and marked bitemporal hemianopia, multiple cranial nerve palsies were present and at the time of examination the tumour was spreading into the orbit and nasopharynx. Classically, from the ophthalmological point of view, chordomas arising in relation to the sella turcica and just lateral to it are the most important, often presenting with chiasmal signs and sixth nerve palsies (Miller, 1972) but the prognosis overall is poor.

Ectopic Pinealoma

Ectopic pinealoma is a very rare tumour occurring in younger age groups, mainly in males and often diagnosed at operation. Classically a pinealoma causes paralysis of upward gaze (Parinaud's syndrome) due to pressure on the colliculi and tectum of the mid-brain. The author has examined one case, a boy aged 12 with bilateral paracentral hemianopic scotomas and Parinaud's syndrome. At operation the tumour was found to have invaded the floor of the third ventricle and impinged on the chiasm posteriorly; following operation the field defects regressed.This experience seems to be in accord with that of Horrax and Wyatt (1947).

Carcinoma

In the author's experience it is rare for metastatic carcinoma to give rise to a chiasmal syndrome but the author has seen one nasopharyngeal carcinoma which presented as a chiasmal syndrome with a right third nerve palsy. However, Thomas and Yoss (1970) in a paper on problems of determining the aetiology of parasellar disease were of the opinion that neoplasia accounted for 70 per cent of all parasellar disease and that of the 70 cases in this category no less than 43 were due to metastatic carcinoma, 50 per cent from nasopharyngeal tumours and the other five per cent from secondary deposits from breast, lung and prostate tumours.

THE EMPTY SELLA SYNDROME

This is a rare syndrome which was originally described in patients who had had chiasmal pressure symptoms and upon surgical exploration were found to have an empty sella (Lee and Adams, 1968). Now the term is also applied to patients in whom chiasmal symptoms recur some years after treatment of the original pituitary tumour. The recrudescence of symptoms in these cases is due to kinking and distortion of the optic nerves and chiasm as they are pulled down into the sella (Obrador, 1972). The author has seen six cases of the empty sella syndrome, all occurring in patients who had had previous treatment for pituitary disease. Four patients had been treated for acromegaly by trans-sphenoidal [90]yttrium implant into the pituitary, one patient had had a chromophobe adenoma removed surgically and the remaining patient had had a chromophobe adenoma treated by external irradiation. All the patients were over 50 years of age and had been treated at least three years previous to the diagnosis of the syndrome being made. One case was explored surgically, the others were diagnosed by air encephalography. All the cases had optic atrophy with increasing field defects which showed, as well as hemianopic defects, constriction of the remaining fields and in two cases upper altitudinal hemianopia. The field defects were steep edged and were adjudged to be vascular in origin. Systemic steroid therapy was given and maintained and none of the patients has subsequently lost fixation, the field defects remaining static. Whether this is a result of the steroid therapy is not known and the arrest of the field defects might well be spontaneous. It is important to remember the eventuality of the empty sella syndrome since, if diagnosed correctly, needless surgery can be avoided. If the field defects progress inexorably, Welch and Stears (1971) advocate the propping up of the chiasm with intrasellar silicone sponge and claim that visual function is improved. If the syndrome is vascular as well as mechanical in origin, this type of therapy would seem to be of very limited application, indeed O'Tenasck and O'Tenasck (1968) reported two cases in which oxidised cellulose used to pack the sella at the time of surgery swelled up post-operatively and caused chiasmal compression.

PREGNANCY AND CHIASMAL DISEASE

It is well known that during pregnancy and subsequently the pituitary gland is enlarged and it has been suggested that a number of pregnant women experience field defects as a result of this enlargement (Finlay, 1934). The author has not found this to be so in normal women but there is no doubt that pregnancy can influence the size of an already existing pituitary tumour, meningioma or vascular tumour. Enoksson, Lundberg and Sjostedts (1961) reported six cases of intracerebral tumours influenced by pregnancy – three suprasellar meningiomas, one craniopharyngioma and two chromophobe adenomas. The author has only seen one such case, a chromophobe adenoma which enlarged during pregnancy causing bitemporal hemianopia but decreased in size following delivery and upon which successful neurosurgery was carried out at a later date. Early in pregnancy it would seem reasonable in such a case to proceed with neurosurgery, while late in pregnancy induction of labour might be called for if vision was threatened by an activated tumour. Pommier and Lafay (1970) have made the point that pregnancy may bring to light an unsuspected pituitary tumour and that in the past such field defects in pregnancy had, at times, been attributed to chiasmal demyelination. More recently it has been suggested that activation of pituitary tumours may be more common in pregnancies which started with an artificially induced ovulation because this is the group in which a small pituitary tumour may have been the cause of selective gonadotrophin insufficiency (Swyer, Little and Harries, 1971). The author has only seen two proven cases of Sheehan's syndrome, neither of whom had any ophthalmological signs of chiasmal dysfunction, which would seem to be in accord with the literature.

OTHER OPHTHALMOLOGICAL ASPECTS OF PITUITARY DISEASE

Retinal pigmentary changes and pituitary disease

The role of the pituitary hormone, melanocyte stimulating hormone (MSH) in relation to the pigment epithelium of the retina is still unknown. There is a possibility that a relationship exists between pituitary disease and the retinal pigment epithelium as evidenced by a number of clinical syndromes in which pituitary disease and retinal pigment degeneration occur, e.g. the Lawrence–Moon–Biedl syndrome. An acromegalic patient has been described in whom, after destruction of the pars intermedia, retinitis pigmentosa developed (Smail, 1972). The author has examined a patient aged 21 who had a chromophobe adenoma of the pituitary removed surgically and then had external irradiation treatment. One year following this he developed a curious superficial pigmentary retinal change in which a reddish-brown pigment appeared in clumps all over both retinae. Electroretinography (ERG) was normal but a fluorogram showed some retinal pigment epithelial migration. In this case an ERG was of the utmost importance in that it ruled out retinitis pigmentosa as the cause for the grouped pigmentary retinal changes.

Pituitary tumours and Marfan's Syndrome

The author has examined two patients with Marfan's syndrome who had pituitary tumours. The first was a 20-year-old female with severe joint changes as a result of Marfan's syndrome and a chromophobe adenoma which was successfully treated surgically. The diagnosis in this case was difficult because of ectopia lentis which made both ophthalmoscopy and field examination difficult. The second case was a 50-year-old female with acromegaly who had been treated with [90]yttrium implantation. She was also an example of Marfan's syndrome. On the basis of two cases no proven relationship between Marfan's syndrome and pituitary tumours can be established but the finding is mentioned in the hope that the situation may be clarified by ophthalmologists being made aware of the possibility.

Pituitary Tumours and Glaucoma

Howard and English (1965) examined 18 acromegalics and the records of a further 52 cases and concluded that there was a 10 per cent incidence of open-angle glaucoma in these cases. This conclusion is of interest for two main reasons: (1) that it may shed some light on the genesis of the glaucomatous process in relation to the pituitary-diencephalic system; and (2) an important consideration in the content of the clinical management and diagnosis of chiasmal disease, glaucomatous cupping of the optic disc could be mistaken for optic atrophy resulting from chiasmal compression and needless neurosurgery carried out. The author has had the opportunity to examine personally 150 cases of acromegaly and the incidence of open angle glaucoma in this series was two per cent. Therefore, while the diagnosis of open angle glaucoma is important, it is rarely a cause for misdiagnosis of chiasmal compression as the incidence would seem to be no greater than in the population at large.

Secondary pituitary hyperplasia

The author has seen two cases of secondary pituitary hyperplasia as the result of long-continued hypothyroidism. This type of hyperplasia has been well recognised but in one of the cases seen, described in full by Richardson and Walsh (1969), some difficulty in precise diagnosis was initially experienced in that a large sella turcica was observed on x-ray and a superior altitudinal field defect was found in one eye. This in fact was due to a uveal effusion which disappeared on thyroxine therapy but illustrates the complexities of some of the clinical diagnoses in pituitary disease.

REFERENCES

Bergland, R. & Ray, B. S. (1969) The arterial supply of the human optic chiasm. *Journal of Neurosurgery,* **31,** 327–334.

Bhagwati, S. N. & Vuckovich, P. M. (1963) Craniopharyngioma presenting with acute blindness. *Archives of Neurology,* **8,** 101.

Blakemore, C. (1970) Binocular depth perception and the optic chiasm. *Vision Research,* **10,** 43–47.

Brougham, M., Heusner, A. P. & Adams, R. D. (1950) Acute degenerative changes in adenomas of the pituitary body with special reference to pituitary apoplexy. *Journal of Neurosurgery,* **7,** 421.

Campbell, A. J. & Ball, J. N. D. (1972) Craniopharyngioma. *Journal of the Canadian Association of Radiologists,* **23,** 182–191.

Crompton, M. R. & Layton, D. P. (1961) Delayed radionecrosis of the brain following therapeutic x-radiation of the pituitary. *Brain,* **84,** 85.

Cullen, J. F., Haining, W. M. & Crombie, A. L. (1966) Cerebral aneurysms presenting with visual field defects. *British Journal of Ophthalmology,* **50,** 251–256.

Cushing, H. (1930) The chiasmal syndrome of primary optic atrophy and bitemporal field defects in adult with a normal sella turcica. *Archives of Ophthalmology* (Chicago), **3,** 505–551.

Dawson, B. H. & Kothandaram, P. (1972) Acute massive infarction of pituitary adenomas. A study of 5 patients. *Journal of Neurosurgery,* **37,** 275–279.

Donin, J. F. (1967) Acquired monocular nystagmus in children. *Canadian Journal of Ophthalmology,* **2,** 212–215.

Elkington, S. G. (1968) Pituitary adenomas. *British Journal of Ophthalmology,* **52,** 322.

Enoksson, P., Lundberg, M. & Sjostedts, S. B. (1961) Influence of pregnancy on visual fields in suprasellar tumours. *Acta Psychiatrica Scandinavica,* **36,** 524-538.

Fein, J. M. & Williams, R. D. B. (1969) See-saw nystagmus. *Journal of Neurology, Neurosurgery and Psychiatry,* **32,** 202-207.

Finlay, C.E. (1934) Bitemporal contraction of visual fields in pregnancy. *Archives of Ophthalmology* (Chicago), **12,** 207–219.

Fisher, N. F., Jampolsky, A. & Scott, A. B. (1968) Traumatic bitemporal haemianopia, Part I. Diagnosis of macular splitting. *American Journal of Ophthalmology,* **65,** 578–581.

Glaser, J. S., Hoyt, W. F. & Corbett, J. (1971) Visual morbidity in chiasmal gliomata. *Archives of Ophthalmology,* **85,** 3–12.

Goldmann, H. (1945) Grundlagen Exacter Perimetric. *Ophthalmologica* (Basel), **109,** 57.

Halliday, A. M., McDonald, W. I. & Mushin, J. (1972) Delayed visual evoked response in optic neuritis. *Lancet,* **i,** 982–985.

Harms, H. (1950) Entwicklungsmogeichkeiten der Perimetric V. Graefe. *Archiv für Ophthalmologie,* **150,** 28.

Hartmann, E., David, M. & Desirgues, P. (1937) Les symptomes oclusive dans les meningiomes olfactifs. *Annales d'Oculistique* (Paris), **174,** 506–527.

Hedges, T. R. (1969) Preservation of the upper nasal field in the chiasmal syndrome, an anatomic explanation. *Transactions of the American Ophthalmological Society,* **67,** 131–141.

Horrax, G. & Wyatt, M. D. (1947) Ectopic pinealomas in the chiasmal region. *Journal of Neurosurgery,* **4,** 309.

Howard, G. M. & English, F. P. (1965) Occurrence of glaucoma in acromegalics. *Archives of Ophthalmology,* **73,** 765–768.

Hoyt, W. F., Sehlicke, B. & Eckethoff, R. J. (1972) Fundoscopic appearance of a nerve fibre bundle defect. *British Journal of Ophthalmology,* **56,** 277–583.

Huber, A. (1961) *Eye Symptoms in Brain Tumours,* pp. 198–202. St Louis: C. V. Mosby.

Jefferson, G. (1940) Extrasellar extension of pituitary adenomas. President's address. *Proceedings of the Royal Society of Medicine,* **33,** 433–458.

Kearns, T. P. & Rucker, C. W. (1957) Arcuate defects in the visual fields due to chromophobe adenoma of the pituitary gland. *American Journal of Ophthalmology,* **45,** 505–507.

Kirkham, T. H. (1972) Hemifield slide phenomenon. *Proceedings of the Royal Society of Medicine,* **65,** 517.

Knight, C. L., Hoyt, W. F. & Wilson, C. B. (1972) Syndrome of prechiasmal optic nerve compression. *Archives of Ophthalmology,* **87,** 1–11.

Lee, W. M. & Adams, J. E. (1968) The empty sella syndrome. *Journal of Neurosurgery,* **28,** 251–356.

Lillie, W. I. (1925) Ocular phenomena in acromegaly. *American Journal of Ophthalmology,* **8,** 32–39.

Lyle, T. K. & Clover, P. (1961) Ocular symptoms and signs in pituitary tumours. *Proceedings of the Royal Society of Medicine,* **54,** 611–619.

Maddox, E. E. (1913) See-saw nystagmus with bi-temporal haemianopia. *Proceedings of the Royal Society of Medicine,* **7,** 12–13.

Matson, D. D. & Crigler, J. F. (1969) Management of craniopharyngioma in childhood. *Journal of Neurosurgery,* **30,** 377–390.

Miller, S. J. H. (1972) Ocular signs of chordomas. *Proceedings of the Royal Society of Medicine*, **65**, 522–523.

Nelson, D. H., Meakins, J. W., Dealy, J. B., Matson, D. D., Emerson, K. & Thorn, G. W. (1958) ACTH producing tumours of the pituitary gland. *New England Journal of Medicine*, **259**, 161–169.

Novotny, H. R. & Alvis, P. L. (1960) A method of photographing fluorescence in circulating blood in the human eye. *American Journal of Ophthalmology*, **50**, 176.

Obrador, S. (1972) The empty sella and some related syndromes. *Journal of Neurosurgery*, **36**, 162–168.

O'Tenasck, F. J. & O'Tenasck, R. J. (1968) Dangers of oxidised cellulose in chiasmal surgery. *Journal of Neurosurgery*, **29**, 209–210.

Pardee, I. H. (1919) Pituitary headaches and their care. *Archives of Internal Medicine* (Chicago), **23**, 174–184.

Pommier, M. L. & Lafay, N. (1970) Syndrome chiasmatique et grosseuse. *Bulletin de la Société d'Ophtalmologie*, **70**, 272–275.

Richardson, J. & Walsh, M. (1969) Uveal effusion as a sign of myxoedema. *British Journal of Ophthalmology*, **53**, 557–560.

Rovit, R. L. & Berry, R. (1965) Cushing's syndrome and the hypophysis, a re-evaluation of pituitary tumours and hyperadrenalism. *Journal of Neurosurgery*, **23**, 270–295.

Russel, D. S. & Rubinstein, L. J. (1963) *Pathology of Tumours of the Nervous System*, pp. 43–58. Baltimore: Williams and Wilkins.

Salassa, R. M., Kearns, T. P., Kernohan, J. W., Sprague, R. G. & MacCarty, C. S. (1959) Pituitary tumours in patients with Cushing's syndrome. *Journal of Clinical Endocrinology*, **19**, 1523–1539.

Schaeffer, J. P. (1924) Some points in the regional anatomy of the optic pathway, with special references to tumours of the hypophysis cerebri and resulting ocular changes. *Anatomical Records*, **28**, 243.

Smail, J. M. (1972) Primary pigmentary degeneration of the retina and acromegaly in a case of pituitary adenoma. *British Journal of Ophthalmology*, **56**, 25–32.

Swyer, G. I. M., Little, V. & Harries, B. J. (1971) Visual disturbance in pregnancy after induction of ovulation. *British Medical Journal*, **iv**, 90–91.

Thomas, J. E. & Yoss, R. E. (1970) Parasellar syndrome, problems in determining aetiology. *Mayo Clinic Proceedings*, **45**, 617–623.

Wagener, H. P. & Cusick, P. L. (1937) Chiasmal syndromes produced by lesions in the posterior fossa. *Archives of Ophthalmology* (Chicago), **18**, 887–891.

Wagener, H. P. & Love, J. G. (1943) Fields of vision in cases of tumours of Rathke's pouch. *Archives of Ophthalmology*, **29**, 873.

Walsh, F. B. & Hoyt, W. F. (1969) *Clinical Neuro-Ophthalmology*, p.2264. Baltimore: Williams and Wilkins.

Welch, K. & Stears, J. C. (1971) Chiasmapexy for the correction of traction on the optic nerves and chiasm. *Journal of Neurosurgery*, **35**, 760–764.

Wilson, P. & Falconer, M. A. (1968) Patterns of visual failure with pituitary tumours. *British Journal of Ophthalmology*, **52**, 94.

Wise, B. L., Brown, H. A., Moffziger, H. C. & Boldreg, E. B. (1955) Pituitary adenomas, carcinoma and craniopharyngioma. *Surgery, Gynaecology and Obstetrics*, **100**, 185.

CHAPTER FIVE

Radiology

M. BANNA

INTERPRETATION OF THE ROUTINE SKULL RADIOGRAPHS

The plain skull radiographs are of the utmost importance in the diagnosis of pituitary lesions. In many cases a definitive diagnosis of a pituitary tumour can be achieved by careful analysis of the plain radiographs.

Routine skull radiographs usually comprise four different views: lateral, postero-anterior, antero-posterior half axial (Towne's view) and a basal view. Additional projections are available as required. These include collimated views of the sella, stereoscopic views and tomograms in the sagittal or the coronal plane. It is essential on examining these films that a systematic search scheme should be adopted by which every structure on the radiograph is carefully examined in respect of the following features:

1. Bony landmarks in the region of the sella for evidence of hyperostosis or bone destruction
2. Presence of calcification within or outside the sella
3. Abnormal vascular markings
4. Delineation and degree of pneumatisation of the sphenoidal sinuses

The lateral skull radiograph (Figure 5.1 a and b)

This is the most informative and often the only diagnostic radiograph. In a good profile projection the two anterior clinoid processes should overlap. This indicates that when the film was taken the mid-sagittal plane of the skull was parallel to the film and that the central x-ray beam was in line with the sella. Slight degrees of rotation can be assessed from the relationship of the anterior clinoid processes and coarser degrees from the relationship of the mandibular rami.

On studying the lateral radiograph, a practical system is to begin by identifying the dense line formed by the compact bone of the planum (jugum) sphenoidale.

Forward continuation of this line leads to the cribriform plate of the ethmoidal bone, whereas its continuation in a posterior direction leads to the following structures from front to back: the limbus sphenoidale (limbus = an edge or border); the inter-optic or chiasmatic sulcus (the groove between the two optic canals); the tuberculum sellae (a small rounded elevation forming the top of the anterior wall of the sella); the lamina dura of the sella and

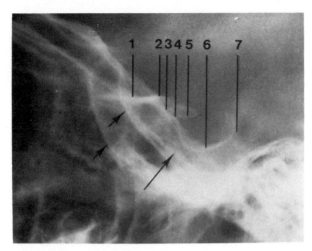

Figure 5.1A. Lateral radiograph of a normal sella. 1 = planum sphenoidale, 2 = Limbus sphenoidale, 3 = sulcus interopticus (chiasmaticus), 4 = tuberculum sellae, 5 = anterior clinoid process, 6 = the lamina dura of the floor of the sella, 7 = the dorsum sellae. The long arrow points to the carotid sulcus. The two short arrows point to the greater wings of the sphenoid bone.

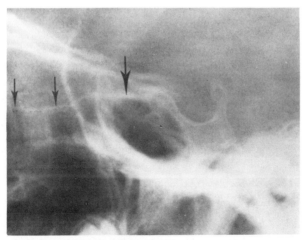

Figure 5.1B. Forward continuation of the line formed by planum sphenoidale (large arrow) leads to the cribriform plate of the ethmoid bone (small arrows).

the dorsum sellae. The posterior clinoid processes are projected over the top of the dorsum sellae and the dense cortical bone of the dorsum can be followed down to the clivus.

Inspection of the lateral radiograph is never complete without examining the sphenoidal sinuses and the retropharyngeal space. This is particularly important if an infrasellar lesion is clinically suspected. The sphenoidal conchae (the thin shell of bone forming the anterior and lower part of the body of the sphenoid bone) is normally obscured by the greater wings of the sphenoid bone but can be easily shown by tomography.

The postero-anterior skull radiograph (Figure 5.2)

In the postero-anterior projection the floor of the sella is projected within the nasal cavity. This radiograph contains considerable information concerning the structures in the neighbourhood of the sella. In identifying these structures it is easier to begin by identifying the dense horizontal line formed by the planum sphenoidale. This line is continuous peripherally with the lesser wings of the sphenoid bone which can be followed outwards to the lateral orbital margin. Beyond that point the lesser wings merge into a thick curved line formed by the fusion of the lesser and greater wings of the sphenoid bone, the frontal and the parietal bones (the pterion). The floor of the sella in this projection lies about one centimetre below and parallel to the planum sphenoidale, varying with the degree of angulation of the x-ray tube.

The medial part of the lesser wing of the sphenoid bone and the anterior clinoid processes form the upper margin of the superior orbital fissure which should then be identified. The inferior boundary to the fissure and the lateral wall of the orbit are formed by the greater wing of the sphenoid bone. Within the outer part of the orbit there is an oblique dense line running from its superior lateral angle downwards and medially. This is a 'shadow line', having no corresponding anatomical structures, and is therefore called the linea innominata. It is formed by that part of the greater wing which is tangential to the x-ray beam. Although our present interest is in the sella, one should not ignore other structures projected on the radiograph as some alterations in these may be the key to the correct diagnosis.

The frontal half-axial skull radiograph (Towne's projection)

With the patient in the supine position and a tube angulation with the orbito-meatal line of approximately 35°, the dorsum sellae is often projected through the foramen magnum. In this projection the dorsum is seen en face, thus enabling destruction limited to one side of the dorsum to be readily detected. It is, however, not always feasible to project the dorsum through the foramen magnum; much depends on the inclination of the skull base and the basal angle.

THE NORMAL SELLA

Variations in the shape of the sella (Figure 5.3)

The shape of the sella on the lateral radiograph differs from one individual to another. It may be circular, oval, bean-shaped or occasionally almost an incomplete square. Usually the antero-posterior diameter of the sella is the largest but the ratio between its length and depth varies and in a deep sella the vertical diameter is the longest diameter of all.

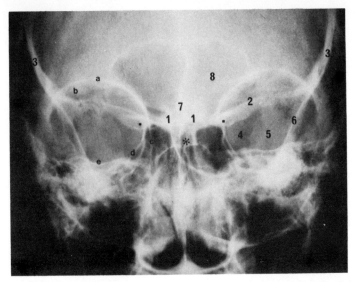

Figure 5.2. Postero-anterior skull radiograph with approximately 15 degrees caudad tilt of the x-ray tube. 1. Planum sphenoidale. 2. Upper anterior margin of the lesser wing of the sphenoid bone. The black dot is on the anterior clinoid process. 3. The bony ridge formed by the fusion of the frontal, parietal and sphenoidal bones. 4. The superior orbital fissure. It transmits to the orbit the oculomotor, trochlear and abducent nerves, the ophthalmic division of the trigeminal nerve, the orbital branch of the middle meningeal artery, and some filaments from the internal carotid plexus of the sympathetic, and from the orbit the ophthalmic veins and a recurrent meningeal artery. 5. The greater wing of the sphenoid bone. 6. Linea innominata. 7. The crista galli. 8. Frontal sinus. a. the orbital roof, b. superior orbital margin, c. anterior portion of the medial wall of the orbit which is mostly formed by the lacrimal bone, d. posterior portion of the medial wall of the orbit. In the absence of any head rotation the distance between c and d should be equal on both sides, e. subarcuate fossa (upper margin of the trigeminal impression). The asterisk marks the place of the pituitary gland and the horizontal line beneath it is the floor of the sella.

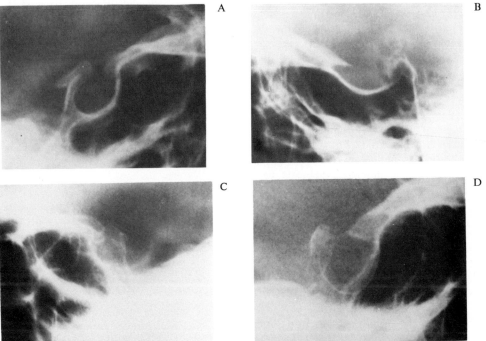

Figure 5.3. Normal variations of the sella in the profile projection. The sella is circular in A, shallow in B, very small in C and deep in D.

Variations of the sulcus interopticus

This is the sulcus between the two optic canals which is commonly known as the sulcus chiasmaticus, although the optic chiasm rarely lies directly above it. Variations in the shape of the sulcus are shown in Figure 5.4. In some individuals no sulcus is present, i.e. there is a straight horizontal line between the planum sphenoidale and the tuberculum sellae. The planum itself is about 1 to 2 mm in thickness and has an even smooth surface. It occasionally ends in a minute bony buttress which should not be confused with hyperostosis due to meningioma, when the new bone formation has an irregular surface.

Variations of the floor of the sella (Figure 5.5)

The floor of the sella is usually formed by a single line of dense cortical bone often called the 'lamina dura'. If the floor is deeper in the centre or if one side is lower than the other a double outline is seen on the lateral radiograph. Rarely, the floor is more uneven and three lines may be seen. These lines are usually 1 to 2 mm apart, each formed of well defined and intact cortical bone joining either anteriorly with the lamina dura, forming the anterior wall of the sella, or posteriorly with the dorsum sellae. In this they differ from a pathological double outline due to unilateral expansion of an intrasellar neoplasm.

Variations of the dorsum sellae

The dorsum sellae is formed by an outer layer of cortical bone and a cancellous inner structure. It shows wide variation in thickness, texture, height and direction. Its anterior cortical layer is usually smooth while the posterior wall is often irregular (Mahmoud, 1958). In children the dorsum is mainly formed of cancellous bone and is short and thick. Its height in adults is about 7 mm and its thickness varies from 2 to 7 mm. The tip of the anterior clinoids, the upper border of the dorsum and the posterior clinoids are usually about the same level.

The dorsum sellae varies in direction; it may rise vertically, slope forwards or it may show a forward concavity. It is thinner in the centre, where it is often saucerised by the pituitary gland, and is thicker peripherally. Because of its shape, the cortical bone in the centre may appear on the lateral radiograph behind the cancellous bone of the thicker outer parts (Figure 5.6), but irrespective of the patient's age or sex, a thin line of lamina dura is always identifiable. Osteoporosis from whatever cause affects mainly the cancellous bone. Thus, even in elderly subjects one can always see, perhaps with the help of a magnifying glass, an intact line of lamina dura.

In some adult subjects the dorsum sellae may be fully pneumatised. Pneumatisation of the sphenoid bone begins in the anterior part of the sinus about the fourth year and gradually extends in a posterior direction, reaching its full size about the age of 20 years (Vidic and Stom, 1968). If the sinus is only partially pneumatised it is its posterior part which remains formed of cancellous bone. A sinus which is opaque anteriorly and translucent posteriorly is pathological.

The infantile sella (Figure 5.7)

Until the seventh or eighth month of intra-uterine life the body of the sphenoid bone consists of two parts; one in front of the tuberculum sellae, forming the presphenoid part

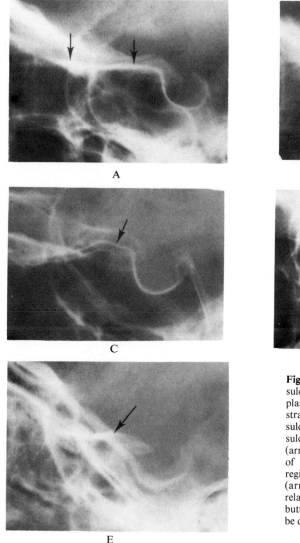

A

C

E

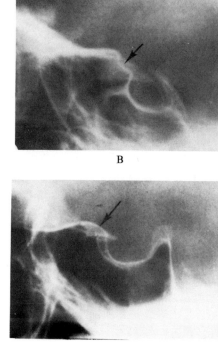

B

D

Figure 5.4. Variations in the shape of the sulcus interopticus (chiasmaticus). A. The planum sphenoidale (arrows) continues as a straight line to the tuberculum sellae. The sulcus interopticus is absent. B. A well-formed sulcus interopticus which is concave in shape (arrow). C. The sulcus interopticus is formed of a straight oblique line (arrow). D. The region of the sulcus is convex in shape (arrow). E. The planum sphenoidale is relatively dense and there is a small bony buttress at the limbus (arrow). This should not be diagnosed as pathological hyperostosis.

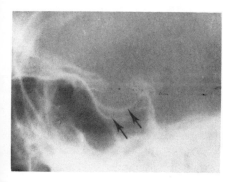

Figure 5.5. Double outline of the sellar floor. This is a normal variation if: 1. the sella is not obviously enlarged, 2. each line of lamina dura is intact, 3. the two lines are no more than 3 mm apart and, 4. they join either anteriorly about the tuberculum sellae or posteriorly at the base of the dorsum.

with which the lesser wings of the sphenoid are continuous; the other comprising the sella turcica and the dorsum sellae, forming the postsphenoid part with which the greater wings are associated. In between these two parts is an oblique translucent cartilaginous cleft known as the intersphenoid or intrasphenoid synchondrosis (Kier, 1968). The presphenoidal and postsphenoidal parts fuse about the eighth month of intra-uterine life but a wedge-shaped piece of cartilage persists for some time and complete ossification does not usually occur before the third postnatal year. Another translucent line which lies behind the intersphenoid synchondrosis, with which it should not be confused, represents the craniopharyngeal canal, and is occasionally visible (Lowman, Robinson and McAllister, 1964). Still more posteriorly there is a third line caused by the spheno-occipital synchondrosis, which is completely fused by the 25th year. In the presence of hydrocephalus the lines of synchondrosis, similar to the suture lines, are wider and their fusion is delayed.

In the period from birth to four years, according to Mahmoud (1958), the sella is shallow, the dorsum sellae is low and the posterior clinoid processes are invisible, since they are not yet ossified. The dorsum increases in height so that the sella becomes deeper, forming about two-thirds of the circumference of a circle at the fourth year. The general outline of the sella does not change perceptibly from the fourth to the 11th year. From the 11th year to maturity, the antero-posterior diameter and the dorsum sellae increase by about one-half to one millimetre each year. From puberty onwards no change takes place in the dimensions of the normal sella.

Variations in the size of the sella

The literature on sellar measurement is voluminous (di Chiro and Nelson, 1962; Oon, 1963), yet like many biological measurements there is a wide range of normal variation which often renders the distinction between a normal and an abnormal sella impossible on measurement alone. We agree with the view put forward by Mahmoud (1958): 'Measurement of the sella turcica is more of academic than clinical significance.'

The methods used for measuring the sella fall into three groups: linear measurements, measurements of the area of the sellar profile and volumetric measurements.

Linear Measurements. The method here described (Figure 5.8) is that devised by Joplin and Fraser (1960) and quoted by Oon (1963). First, a line between the nasion and the tuberculum sellae is drawn for orientation. The length of the sella turcica is then measured as the greatest antero-posterior diameter parallel to that line. The depth is the longest perpendicular line from the sellar floor to a line joining the tuberculum and the most anterior convexity of the posterior clinoids. These measurements as stated by Oon (1963) are: antero-posterior diameter varies from 8 to 15 mm (mean 11.3); vertical diameter varies from 6.5 to 12.5 mm (mean 8.9).

Measurement of the area of the sellar profile. The most accurate measurement is probably that of Mahmoud (1958) using a planimeter. It is of little practical value, however, and once again the normal variation is extremely wide ranging from 20 to 130 mm^2.

Measurement of the sellar volume. For measuring the volume of the sella, di Chiro and Nelson (1962) devised the following equation and found that the sellar volume varies from 240 mm^3 to 1092 mm^3 (mean 594 mm^3):

Sellar volume $= \frac{1}{2}$ length $\times$ depth $\times$ width

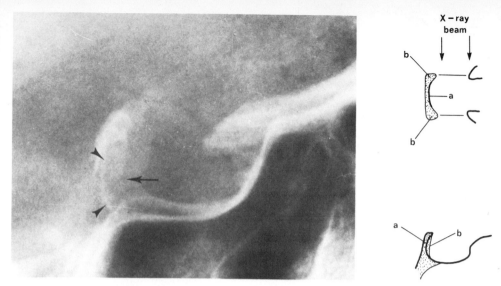

Figure 5.6. A magnified view of a normal sella. In this case the cortical bone in the centre of the dorsum (arrow heads on the radiograph and letter 'a' on the diagram) is projected behind the cancellous bone in its periphery (single arrow on the radiograph and letter 'b' on the diagram).

A B

C D

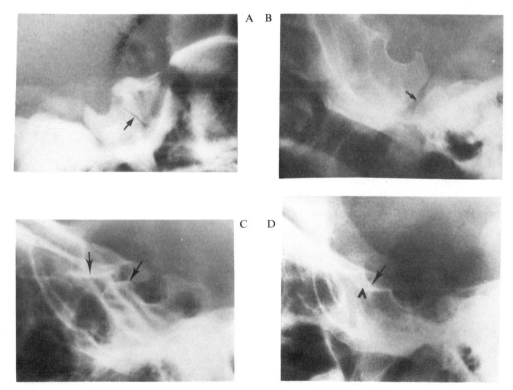

Figure 5.7. Some observations on the infantile sella. A. A 32 week premature infant. Arrow points at intersphenoid synchondrosis which separates the presphenoidal from the postsphenoidal part of the sphenoid bone. This line usually disappears within the first postnatal year and no later than the third year. It is wider in the presence of hydrocephalus. B. Arrow points at the spheno-occipital synchrondrosis which ossifies completely by about the twenty-fifth year. C. The discontinuity of the lamina dura between the two arrows is due to the non-ossified cartilaginous limbus sphenoidale. In older children a notch is frequently present at this site prior to union of the limbus to the presphenoid. D. Arrow points to a prominent roof of the optic canal, appearing as a false excavation. This appearance is accentuated on an imperfect lateral radiograph. It should not be described as a J-shaped sella. On careful inspection a normal planum can be seen (arrow head).

The sellar length equals the greatest horizontal antero-posterior diameter.

For measuring the sellar depth a line is first drawn between the tuberculum sellae and the top of the dorsum. The depth of the sella equals the height of a perpendicular to that line drawn from the deepest point in the floor of the sella. If there are two contours of the floor a mid-point between them is taken for measurement. Evaluation of the sellar width may be obtained from:

1. The width of the dorsum sella at its narrowest point, the 'waist' of the dorsum, as seen in the half axial projection.
2. The floor of the sella on the straight postero-anterior or antero-posterior radiographs, or in doubtful cases on coronal plane tomograms.
3. The anterior or the posterior walls of the sella as seen on the submento-vertical projection. These two lines are, however, often difficult to identify.

It should be pointed out that all previous measurements were made on conventional radiographs with a tube film distance of 90 to 100 cm. This gives a magnification factor of about 15 per cent. Using tomograms, a magnification factor of up to 40 per cent may be present. If the focal film distance is shorter than 90 cm or if the x-ray film is moved away from the skull, the above measurements are invalid.

Ligamentous calcification around the sella (Figure 5.9)

Physiological calcification in the interclinoid or petroclinoid ligaments is common and it has no pathological significance. It may be unilateral or bilateral and may lead to a 'bridged sella'. This type of calcification appears on the lateral radiograph as if it were within the sella, but as it lies on the sides of the pituitary gland it is never a cause of pituitary dysfunction.

The J-shaped sella

The range of what this term implies varies from a normal, perhaps somewhat deep, concave chiasmatic sulcus on the one hand to deeply excavated and obviously eroded anterior clinoid processes on the other. In both conditions the sella simulates the letter J lying on its side. Other descriptive terms which are in use include: pear-shaped, omega-shaped, shoe-shaped and hour-glass sella. Using any of these adjectives on their own may not convey to the reader what the observer means. There are numerous conditions in which a J-shaped sella may be seen. These include five per cent of normal children, a fewer number of normal adults, bone dysplasia, gargoylism, achondroplasia, osteogenesis imperfecta, mongolism, neurofibromatosis, chronic hydrocephalus, craniopharyngioma, suprasellar dermoid and optic chiasm glioma (Burrows, 1964). It has also been shown that a tilted lateral radiograph of a normal skull in a child may, due to elevation of the floor of the laterally positioned optic canal, result in a J-shaped sella (Kier, 1968). We are of the opinion that such a purely descriptive term should not be used without further elucidation of its significance.

CALCIFICATION IN THE SELLAR REGION

Physiological calcification occurring in the ligaments around the sella has been described above. Any other type of calcification occurring in this area is pathological but its significance varies; for instance, atheromatous calcification in the internal carotid artery is a fairly common finding in elderly subjects and can be readily recognised from its shape,

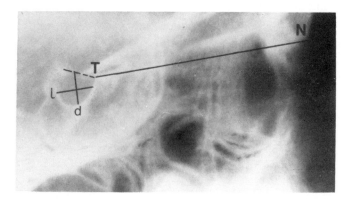

Figure 5.8. Sellar measurement as proposed by Joplin and Fraser (1960). Prior to measurement draw a line from the nasion to the tuberculum (NT) for orientation. The length of the sella (L) is the greatest fossa diameter parallel to the NT line. The depth (d) is the greatest distance (perpendicular to the length) from the sellar floor to a line joining the tuberculum and the most anterior convexity of the posterior clinoids.

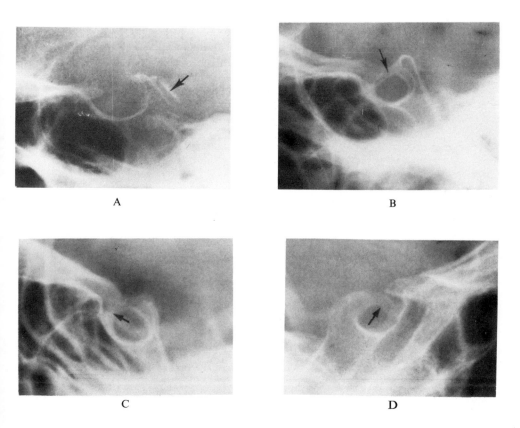

Figure 5.9. Ligamentous calcification around the sella. A. Calcification of petro-clinoid ligaments. B. Calcification of the ligaments between the anterior and posterior clinoids. C. calcification in the ligament between the anterior and middle clinoid processes, producing a caroticlinoid foramen for the internal carotid artery. D. Calcification between the middle and posterior clinoids.

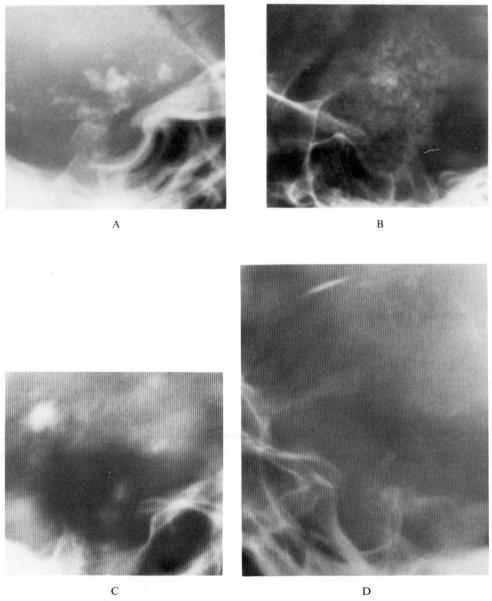

Figure 5.10. These lateral radiographs belong to four patients with different lesions. It is evident that on the basis of radiographic appearances alone it is impossible to predict the nature of the lesion. A. Multiple calcified tuberculomas. B. Hypothalamic glioma (By courtesy of Dr E. H. Burrows and the Editors of the *British Journal of Radiology*). C. Craniopharyngioma. D. Cholesteatoma.

both on the lateral and antero-posterior radiographs. Similarly nodular calcification in a patient with a past history of tuberculous meningitis should present no problem.

Neoplastic calcification occurs in a large variety of tumours which include craniopharyngioma, pituitary adenoma, meningioma, glioma, angioma, chordoma, teratoma and infundibuloma but on morphological grounds alone, it is impossible to ascribe any type of calcification to a particular lesion (Figure 5.10). The patient's age, the clinical manifestations, the type of sellar changes, the presence of bone sclerosis or destruction are all valuable in forming a specific pathological diagnosis. However, sometimes the pathological diagnosis may not be clear until exploration.

Among tumours of the sellar region, craniopharyngioma has the highest incidence of calcification and since this tumour is more common in children, any suprasellar calcification in a child is highly suggestive of this tumour. Other causes of suprasellar calcification in childhood are rare.

The majority of tumours, other than craniopharyngioma, occur in adults and in them chromophobe adenoma is the commonest. Only a minority of these tumours show radiological evidence of calcification which may be nodular within the tumour substance or curvilinear occurring in the tumour capsule. The latter gives the impression that it is in the wall of a cystic lesion. In the presence of curvilinear calcification differentiation between a solid and a cystic tumour may be possible on brain scintigraphy (Figure 5.11). A solid tumour is more likely to show a high uptake whereas a cystic lesion (with the exception of an aneurysm) usually gives a normal brain scintigram. Calcification in meningioma is usually associated with hyperostosis and only rarely is this tumour accompanied by bone

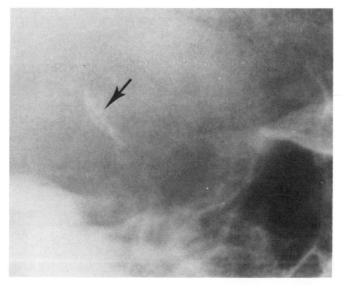

Figure 5.11. Calcification in the capsule of chromophobe adenoma. This is rare and often diagnosed as cystic craniopharyngioma, especially when the main enlargement of the sella is in its outlet, as in this case. The brain scintigram (Tc 99m) seen below suggested that the tumour was solid. It was later revealed to be a chromophobe adenoma. Thus, in the presence of cystic type of calcification and high uptake of the radioactive isotope, the lesion is most likely a chromophobe adenoma. (By kind permission of the editor of *Journal of the Neurological Sciences.*)

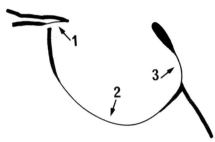

Figure 5.12A. 'Ballooning' of the sella from an intrasellar tumour. Note: 1. undermining of the anterior clinoids; 2. erosion of the sellar floor: 3. thinning of the dorsum sellae. The posterior clinoids are preserved and may be carried upwards on the surface of the tumour.

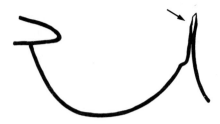

Figure 5.12B. Widening of the sellar outlet by a suprasellar tumour. Note: The direction of dislocation of the dorsum and early erosion of the posterior clinoids.

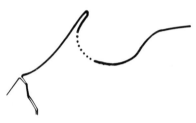

Stage I. Erosion (indicated by the dotted line) of the lamina dura of the base of the dorsum sellae and the posterior portion of the floor of the sella.

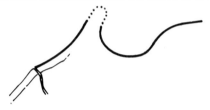

Stage II (a). Erosion of the posterior clinoids and the top of the dorsum sellae.

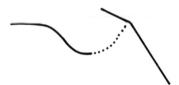

Stage II (b). Thinning of the dorsum sellae which may be also dislocated by an enlarged or a depressed third ventricle.

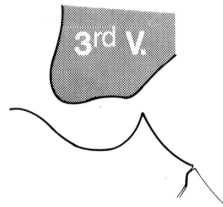

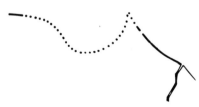

Stage III. The dorsum sellae may gradually disappear and complete resorption of the floor of the sella may occur. Rarely, this bone resorption extends forwards to the planum sphenoidale and may even involve the floor of the anterior cranial fossa.

Stage IV. Widening of the sellar outlet with varying degree of bone resorption which may be limited to the dorsum. This type of sellar change is more liable to occur in chronic obstructive hydrocephalus such as in aqueduct stenosis. Here the dilated third ventricle may herniate through the diaphragma sellae compressing the pituitary gland and occupying a large space within the sella.

Figure 5.13. Sellar changes due to raised intracranial pressure.

destruction, this being more frequently seen with chordoma. Calcification in a chordoma may have a multicystic appearance due to the mucin content of the tumour, in which case it may be difficult to differentiate from an osteochondroma arising in the skull base. Calcification in a hypothalamic glioma is exceedingly rare and is indistinguishable from that occurring in craniopharyngioma. The same is true of calcification in infundibuloma.

One type of pituitary calcification may be seen as an incidental finding in the elderly. This consists of a small intrasellar calcification about 5 mm in diameter occurring in an inactive pituitary adenoma. This type of lesion has been described as 'pituitary calculus' (Mascherpa and Valentino, 1959).

SELLAR CHANGES DUE TO PITUITARY AND PARAPITUITARY TUMOURS

In the following paragraphs only the classical appearances of these tumours will be considered and these will not be seen in every case. Variations are by no means rare since a tumour arising primarily above the sella may extend into the confines of the sella and a sellar tumour with a small intrasellar component may expand primarily in an upward direction. In an entirely intrasellar tumour the main sellar changes are (Figure 5.12A):
1. Uniform expansion or 'ballooning' of the sella.
2. Undermining of the anterior clinoid processes.
3. Thinning of the dorsum sellae due to excavation by the tumour. The dorsum later may be completely destroyed but the posterior clinoid processes are usually preserved. They may be displaced upwards on the surface of the tumour.
4. Thinning of the floor of the sella which may later be destroyed leading to a soft tissue shadow of the tumour projecting into the sphenoidal air sinus.
   In an entirely suprasellar tumour the following changes may be seen (Figure 5.12B):
1. Widening of the outlet of the sella.
2. Erosion of the posterior clinoids and the top of the dorsum sellae. The floor of the sella remains intact and undermining of the anterior clinoids is not a feature of suprasellar tumours.
   Retrosellar tumours may lead to destruction of the posterior wall of the dorsum sellae and of the clivus, which may extend at a later stage to involve other structures in the base of the skull.
   Infrasellar tumours (in their early stages) may cause destruction of the sphenoidal air sinus and the floor of the sella and may be accompanied by a retropharyngeal soft tissue swelling.

THE SELLA IN RAISED INTRACRANIAL PRESSURE

The development of the radiological changes occurring in the sella turcica as a result of increased intracranial pressure can be divided into the following four stages (Figure 5.13).

Stage I: Erosion of the lamina dura in the anterior part of the base of the dorsum sellae

This is an early radiological manifestation of raised intracranial pressure and is estimated to occur five to six weeks from its onset. Although it is characteristic of raised intracranial pressure, similar changes have been reported in about seven per cent of patients suffering from systemic arterial hypertension (Fry and du Boulay, 1965).

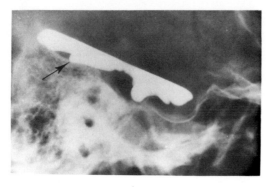

A

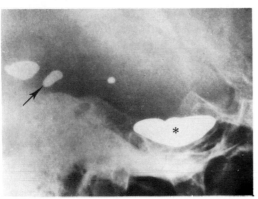

B

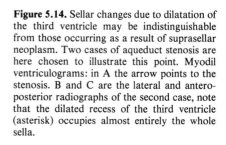

Figure 5.14. Sellar changes due to dilatation of the third ventricle may be indistinguishable from those occurring as a result of suprasellar neoplasm. Two cases of aqueduct stenosis are here chosen to illustrate this point. Myodil ventriculograms: in A the arrow points to the stenosis. B and C are the lateral and antero-posterior radiographs of the second case, note that the dilated recess of the third ventricle (asterisk) occupies almost entirely the whole sella.

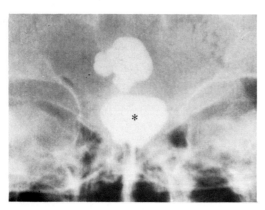

C

Stage II: Erosion of the posterior clinoids and the top of the dorsum sellae

The change described as Stage I has progressed and as a result of further erosion the dorsum is shortened. Shortening of the dorsum may also occur as a result of direct pressure from a dilated third ventricle acting as a suprasellar tumour.

Stage III: Complete absorption of the lamina dura of the sella and the dorsum sellae

This occurs in more chronic cases and the bone resorption may extend forward as far as the planum sphenoidale.

Stage IV: A long shallow sella without any visible dorsum

This occurs in chronic obstructive hydrocephalus such as in cases of aqueduct stenosis. The dilated anterior recesses of the third ventricle may extend into the pituitary fossa compressing the gland (Figure 5.14).

Sellar changes simulating those due to increased intracranial pressure may be seen with pituitary adenoma and the distinction between these two conditions on radiological grounds alone may be impossible (Figure 5.15). It is equally difficult, when only the top of the dorsum is eroded or the outlet of the sella is enlarged, to distinguish between cases due to dilatation of the third ventricle and others due to suprasellar neoplasm unless one takes into consideration the clinical picture and other radiological changes that may be present in the tumour cases.

In children the main feature of raised intracranial pressure is suture diastasis. This may occur with or without sellar changes depending on the child's age. In children less than six or seven years of age suture diastasis is frequently the only sign of raised intracranial pressure. In this age group separation of sutures occurs very early during the first few days or weeks of the condition. Erosion of the sella turcica without any suture diastasis at this age is nearly always an indication of local erosion by a tumour such as a craniopharyngioma or an optic chiasm glioma. From seven until about ten years, in addition to suture diastasis, the sella is also affected more often than not, so that both these signs of raised intracranial pressure are present although the diastasis may be more obvious and the sellar changes may be overlooked. After the tenth birthday, destruction of the sella is somewhat more commonly seen as the only evidence of raised intracranial pressure (du Boulay, 1957). According to Bull (1953), suture diastasis is rare over the age of ten, very rare indeed over 15 and practically non-existent over the age of 20. After the closure of sutures – that is after about the age of 10 years – suture diastasis is hardly ever seen until the intracranial pressure has been raised for many months, and in these older children it may serve as confirmation that the condition is a long standing one (du Boulay, 1957).

Although the majority of cases having radiological evidence of raised intracranial pressure may have headaches, vomiting or papilloedema, this is by no means universal. Exceptions are common, particularly in younger children with slowly growing tumours in whom enlargement of the head is tantamount to a partial decompression. Even in adults the sellar changes may occur in the absence of papilloedema, partly due to the fact that the extension of the subarachnoid space along the optic nerves varies and may not extend as far as the eyeball. du Boulay and El-Gammal (1966), in a review study of a large number of intracranial tumours, pointed out that one-fifth of their cases, with evident sellar changes, were without definite evidence of papilloedema.

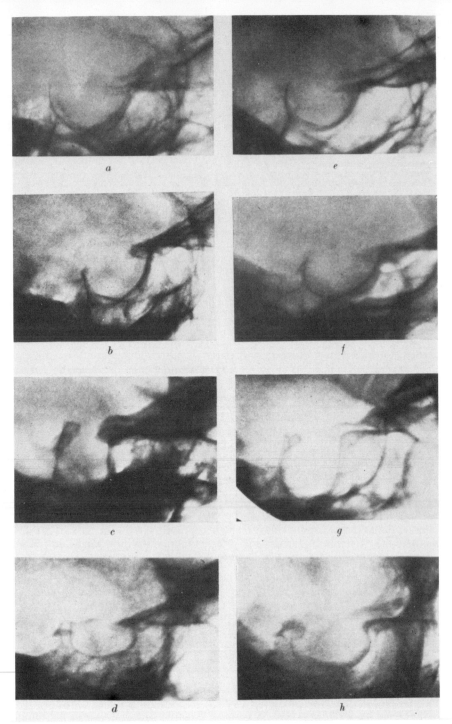

Figure 5.15. Lateral view of sella turcica in eight different cases, two of which are always extraordinarily alike. In each pair, however, one shows a pituitary tumour, and the other excavation of the sella due to an increase in intracranial pressure. The former are the cases A to D, the latter the case E to H. In none of the cases is there any doubt that pathological changes have occurred at the sella turcica. In spite of this, differential diagnosis is not possible on the basis of the appearance of the sella turcica alone. Although such similarities are rare in obviously pathological cases, it becomes apparent that in borderline cases, differential diagnosis is even more difficult. (After the late Professor E. G. Mayer (1959) and by kind permission of Springer-Verlag, Wien.)

CEREBRAL ANGIOGRAPHY

In this section three topics will be discussed: the basic radiographic appearances of a normal carotid angiogram, the value of cerebral angiography in the diagnosis of pituitary and parapituitary tumours and the findings which may be seen if such a lesion is present.

The normal carotid angiogram

As routine films in the arterial, the capillary and the venous phases of the cerebral circulation are obtained the most useful views for pituitary lesions are the lateral and antero-posterior radiographs without tube tilt. The main vessels are shown in Figure 5.16 – A, B and C.

The value of cerebral angiography in the diagnosis of pituitary tumours

1. To exclude an aneurysm which may be present as the primary lesion or rarely in association with a pituitary neoplasm. This incidental association was seen twice during the present study and its effects on management are important.
2. To illustrate the anatomical relationships of the tumour to the neighbouring vessels.
3. To attempt to achieve a pre-operative pathological diagnosis, but as will be seen later in the description of the radiographic appearances of specific tumours, only a small number show evidence of pathological circulation on the conventional angiogram.
4. To assess the size of the cerebral ventricles.

Information about ventricular size may influence the choice between air encephalography and ventriculography as the next investigation and this information may be obtained by consideration of:

1. The shape of the sweep of the pericallosal artery (Figure 5.17). Elevation of the pericallosal artery requires a moderate degree of ventricular dilatation before it can be recognised with certainty on the angiogram. This is because the artery lies above the superior medial angle of the ventricle which is altered only at a late stage of the ventricular dilatation.
2. The shape of the thalamo-striate vein on the antero-posterior radiograph is the most accurate index of ventricular size (Figure 5.18). The vein lies on the infero-lateral wall of the lateral ventricle and is pushed outwards and downwards as the ventricle dilates.
3. The avascularity of the cerebral ventricles may sometimes be clearly distinguished in films recording the capillary phase of the cerebral circulation.
4. In severe degrees of ventricular dilatation there is widening of the U-shaped space between the anterior and middle cerebral arteries, elevation of the Sylvian vessels and stretching of the deep cerebral veins.

The angiographic findings in pituitary and parapituitary tumours

Elevation of the horizontal segment of the anterior cerebral artery on the antero-posterior radiograph is the most common abnormality (Figure 5.19). In normal individuals this segment runs a more or less horizontal course but may be inclined slightly upwards or markedly downwards depending on the tortuosity of the vessel and on the x-ray tube angulation (Krayenbühl and Yasargil, 1968). In its course towards the midline, the anterior cerebral artery may follow either a direct horizontal course or it may be directed forward

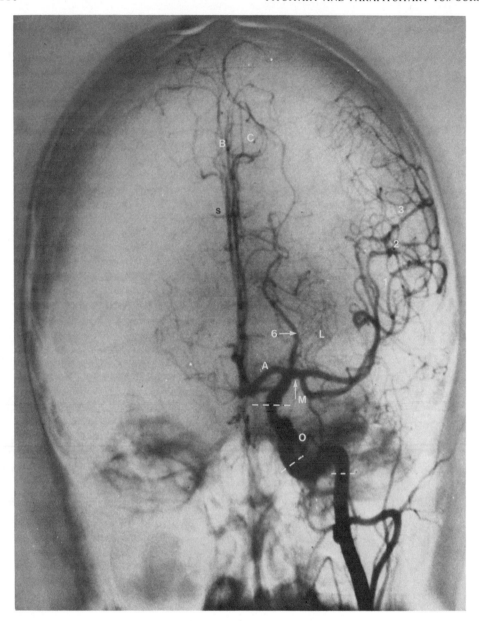

A

Figure 5.16A and B. Arterial phase of normal carotid angiogram (antero-posterior and lateral radiographs). *The internal carotid artery* is anatomically divided into four portions (dotted lines): cervical, petrous, cavernous and cerebral. The latter gives rise to the ophthalmic artery (0), the posterior communicating artery (P) connecting with the posterior cerebral artery (6) and the anterior choroidal artery (7). *The anterior cerebral artery* divides into two main branches; the pericallosal (B) and the callosomarginal (C). Other named branches are frontopolar artery (D), the orbital branches (E) and artery of the cingulate gyrus (s, on the anterior radiograph). *The middle cerebral artery.* This artery divides first into two or three main vessels from which four branches or sub-branches can usually be recognised: ascending fronto-parietal (1), parietal (2), angular (3) and posterior temporal artery (4). A fifth small branch, the anterior temporal artery (5) is occasionally identified. The lenticulostriate arteries are best seen on the antero-posterior view (L).

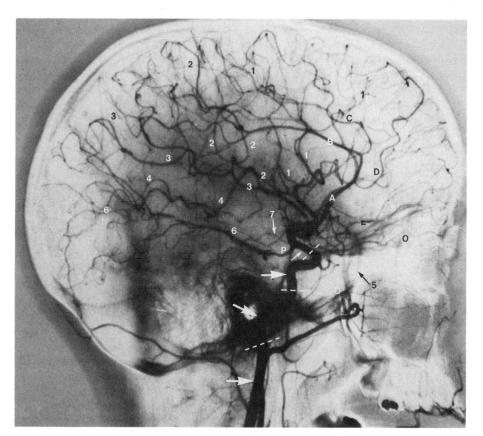

B

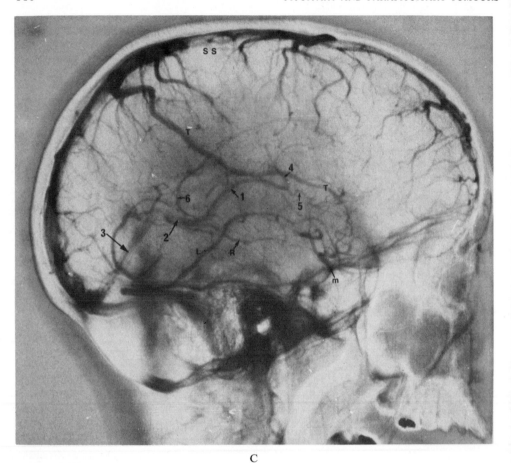

C

Figure 5.16C. The venous phase of normal carotid angiogram. The cerebral veins are divisable into two groups: a superficial or cortical and a deep or internal group. The cortical veins drain mainly into the superior sagittal sinus (SS) through the superior cortical veins. The inferior cortical veins are smaller and fewer and they drain into the middle cerebral vein and the dural sinuses in the skull base. The number and the configuration of the superficial veins is very variable.

The deep cerebral veins are constant though some variation in their shape does exist between different individuals. They are formed by two internal veins (1), one in each hemisphere, which unite to form the great cerebral vein or the vein of Galen (2). This drains into the straight sinus (3). There are many tributaries to the internal cerebral vein and they include: the thalamostriate vein (4), the septal vein (5), the posterior callosal vein (6) and the basal vein of Rosenthal (R). The venous angle is formed by the junction thalamostriate vein with the internal cerebral vein. Two anastomotic veins are usually present: a superior anastomotic vein or vein of Trolard (T) draining into the superior sagittal sinus and an inferior anastomotic vein or vein of Labbé (L) ending into the lateral sinus.

and medially (Gado and Bull, 1971). Thus the degree of elevation by a suprasellar tumour depends not only on the size and site of the tumour but also on the anatomical course of the vessel as it is less likely to be distorted if it is running in a forward and medial direction. However, the shape of the vessel on the antero-posterior radiograph may be misleading. When the point of bifurcation of the internal carotid artery is elevated, the anterior cerebral artery, despite its elevation, may appear horizontal on the antero-posterior radiograph. This error can be avoided by assessing the shape of the carotid siphon on the lateral projection. The second most important feature of parasellar tumours is distortion of the cavernous portion of the internal carotid artery (Bull and Schunk, 1962) (Figure 5.20).

Other types of vascular displacements which are not characteristic of, but may be seen with large suprasellar tumours include lateral displacement of the anterior choroidal arteries and the striatal arteries (Figure 5.21) and elevation of the internal cerebral veins and the venous angle which abuts on the posterior margin of the foramen of Monro and when displaced indicates a large tumour possibly leading to hydrocephalus (Figure 5.22).

CEREBRAL PNEUMOGRAPHY

The outline of the cerebral ventricles can be revealed radiographically by the introduction of contrast media either directly into the ventricles (ventriculography), or indirectly through the lumbar subarachnoid space (lumbar air encephalography or pneumoencephalography). The latter is the examination of choice for the investigation of pituitary and parapituitary tumours because it outlines the basal cisterns as well as the ventricles, but lumbar introduction of air is contra-indicated in the presence of clinical or radiological evidence of raised intracranial pressure. In these cases, ventriculography is considered a safer procedure. There are, however, cases in which, following ventriculography, pneumoencephalography is required to outline the basal cisterns. Under these circumstances, the examination should be carried out in full liaison with a neurosurgeon who should be prepared to undertake immediate surgical treatment if indicated.

Air is the contrast medium most commonly used for pneumoencephalography and ventriculography. Some investigators prefer to use oxygen because of its more rapid absorption and the avoidance of the very small risk of air embolism. We do not find rapid absorption a major advantage and have used air in all our cases except in children where there is said to be a greater risk of air embolism because of the small blood volume compared to the volume of air needed to demonstrate the cerebral ventricles. The air should be fractioned, i.e. injecting 8 to 10 ml at a time. The total amount required depends on the size of the ventricles, bearing in mind that the average normal ventricular system has a capacity of less than 20 ml, probably about 16 ml. Various authors have recommended different volumes of cerebrospinal fluid withdrawal but all agree that the total volume of air injected should be larger than the cerebrospinal fluid withdrawn.

This conclusion is based on the observation that the increase of cerebrospinal fluid pressure following the air injection is only of short duration, much shorter than the time necessary for a decreased cerebrospinal fluid pressure to return to normal values. A transient hypertension in the subarachnoid space is considered to be less dangerous than a prolonged hypotension (Ruggiero, 1966). In general, sufficient air should be introduced to fill half the body of the lateral ventricle, thus the combined radiographs taken in the brow-up and the brow-down positions will outline the whole ventricular system. Where there is severe ventricular dilatation requiring more than 50 ml of air, it is safer to use a positive contrast medium, thus avoiding pressure changes which could precipitate brain herniation or subdural haematoma. Approximately 3 ml of ethyl iodophenylundecanoate (Myodil) are

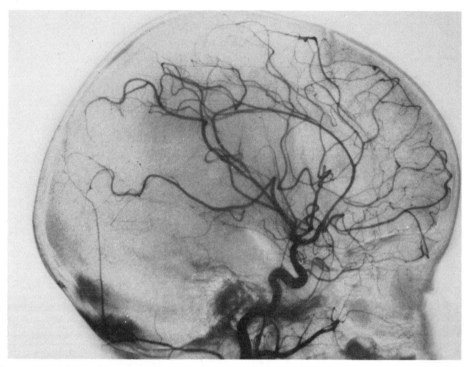

Figure 5.17. Widening of the sweep of the pericallosal artery due to moderate ventricular dilatation.

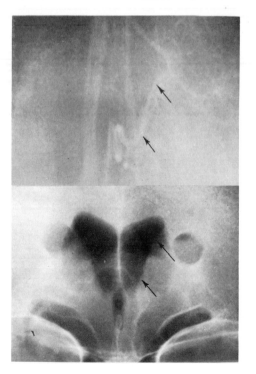

Figure 5.18. The shape of the thalamo-striate vein on the antero-posterior radiograph provides the most accurate angiographic index of ventricular size. The arrows in the top picture point to the thalamo-striate vein. The arrows in the bottom picture point at the impression formed by the head of the caudate nucleus where the vein lies. Both illustrations are of the same patient. The small illustration (below right) shows the shape of the vein in a case of ventricular dilatation.

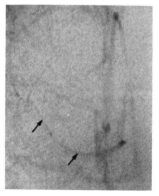

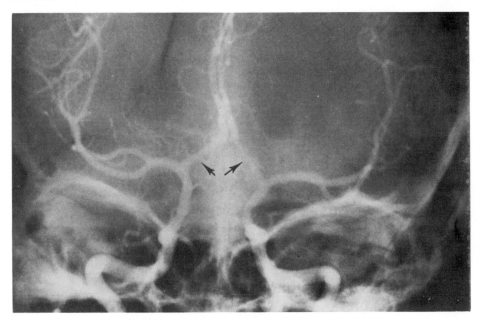

Figure 5.19. Upward displacement of the horizontal segment of the anterior cerebral arteries.

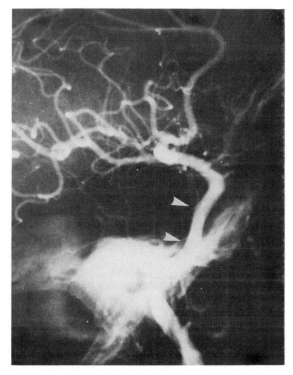

Figure 5.20A. Forward displacement of the cavernous part of the internal carotid artery (arrow) by a large chromophobe adenoma.

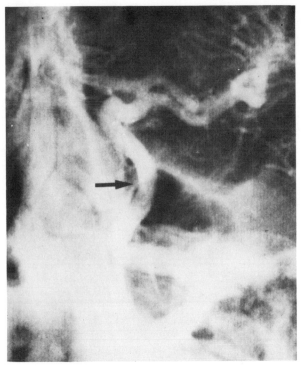

Figure 5.20B. Lateral displacement of the cavernous part of the internal carotid artery (arrow) by a chromophobe adenoma. As incidental finding note that at the carotid bifurcation the middle cerebral artery arises as two separate vessels, i.e. there is an accessory middle cerebral artery (an anatomical variant).

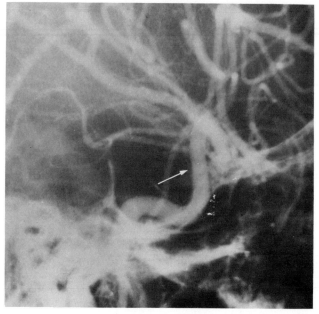

Figure 5.20C. Upward and forward displacement of the distal limb of the carotid siphon from a craniopharyngioma.

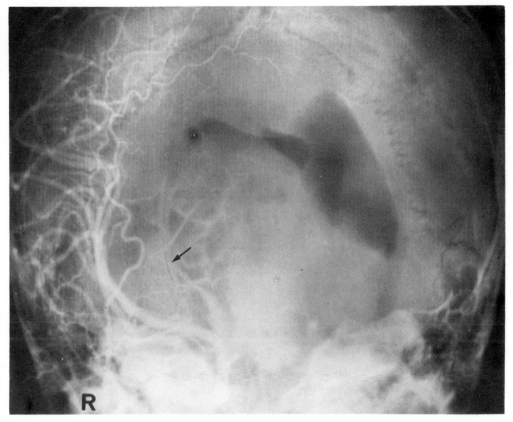

Figure 5.21. Stretching and lateral displacement of the striatal branches by a large craniopharyngioma.

introduced into the frontal horn of one lateral ventricle, preferably in the non-dominant hemisphere. The head is then manipulated under fluoroscopic control, so as to direct the Myodil into the third ventricle. A water soluble contrast medium, either meglumine iothalamate (Conray 60) or meglumine iocarmate (Dimer X), has been used for ventriculography in some centres. This type of contrast medium has not yet been accepted as absolutely safe. It has been tried in few cases in our clinic but we are not yet in a position to recommend its general use or role. The radiological anatomy relevant to pituitary tumours is shown in Figures 5.23 and 24.

THE RADIOLOGICAL CHANGES DUE TO PITUITARY ADENOMA

The classical radiological changes due to pituitary adenoma are those of an intrasellar tumour described on page 111.

As might be expected, not every case is typical and in order to acquaint the reader with the variety of sellar changes he is likely to encounter, we have illustrated 12 examples from a series of sixty chromophobe adenomas emphasising the main features (Figure 5.25). One notices that in many of these illustrations (Figures c, d, e, f, i and j) the diagnosis of a pituitary adenoma is easy, but in some, as in Figures h and l, the changes are atypical. Furthermore, where the sella and the dorsum sellae are destroyed, as in Figure 5.25 k, it is difficult to know the origin of the tumour. In Figures 5.25 a and b, the sella is not enlarged and the changes are subtle. Such infrequent cases without sellar enlargement may even be accompanied by a large suprasellar extension. According to Ambrose (1973): 'between 5 and 10 per cent of chromophobe adenomas do not produce any significant enlargement of the sella and it is probable that the aperture in the diaphragma sellae in these cases is large, allowing tumour to escape the confines of the sella. On the other hand, if the aperture is small the enlargement of the sella in a downward direction may be extensive.' It is in this relatively small percentage of cases that tomography in the sagittal and coronal planes is informative.

Occasionally the sella changes from pituitary adenoma closely mimic those resulting from increased intracranial tension, so that differentiation on radiological grounds alone is almost impossible (Figure 5.15). Less frequently in cases of pituitary adenoma, one may find that it is mainly the outlet of the sella which is widened; an appearance which is more representative of suprasellar than intrasellar neoplasm. In such a case, only a small portion of the tumour is intrasellar, the larger portion being above the sella.

Histological evidence of calcification in chromophobe adenoma is not uncommon, but it is seldom dense enough to cast a shadow on the skull radiograph. The incidence of radiologically visible calcification in our series was four per cent but it varies in different reports from one to six per cent (du Boulay and Trickey, 1962). Calcification may be granular or nodular when it occurs within the tumour substance or curvilinear when developing in the tumour capsule (Figures 5.26 and 5.11).

The sellar changes due to an eosinophilic adenoma are similar to those associated with the chromophobe type and there is no single feature in a specific case that permits differentiation (Figure 5.27). However, in analysing a large series of cases the balloon-shaped sella is predominantly found in eosinophilic adenomas. By contrast in chromophobe adenomas, the sella is more often cup-shaped and there is a higher incidence of destruction of the dorsum sellae and asymmetry of the floor of the sella (Ross and Greitz, 1966).

Systemic changes due to eosinophilic pituitary adenoma

The overproduction of the somatotrophic hormone, whether due to an eosinophilic adenoma, a mixed tumour, or to hyperplasia of the eosinophilic cells without adenomatous formation, leads to an excessive growth of all connective tissue, cartilage and bone. Thus, there is increased thickness of the skin, hypertrophy of the tongue, mild generalised enlargement of the liver, kidneys and spleen, mild swelling of the joints due to excessive proliferation of cartilage and thickening of ligaments, bursae and synovial membranes. Excessive growth of the skeletal tissue before epiphyseal closure leads to increased length of the tubular bones and possibly to gigantism. As the disease usually occurs in patients already past puberty, increase in height is uncommon but in this age group cartilagenous proliferation and ossification may continue to occur, resulting in a wide range of radiological abnormalities (Steinbach, Feldman and Goldberg, 1959).

In the skull there is thickening of the vault and increased bone density leading to loss of definition between diploe and compact bone and excessive hyperostosis interna. There is enlargement of all paranasal sinuses, most obvious in the frontal bone and proliferation of the mastoid air cells. The frontal sinus is said to be abnormally large in about 50 per cent of males and 25 per cent of female acromegalics and this is believed to be the result of

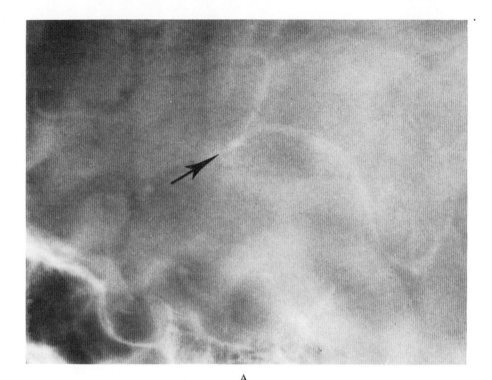

A

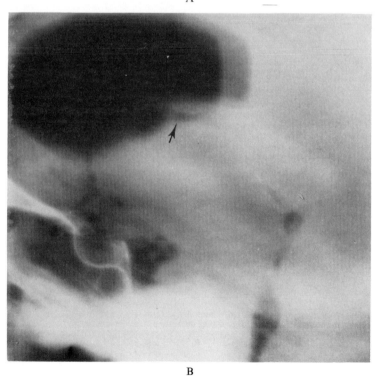

B

Figure 5.22. A. Venous phase of the carotid angiogram. The internal cerebral vein is elevated and the venous angle (arrow) is posteriorly displaced by a large suprasellar tumour shown at pneumoencephalography (B) where the third ventricle (arrow) aqueduct and fourth ventricle are all displaced.

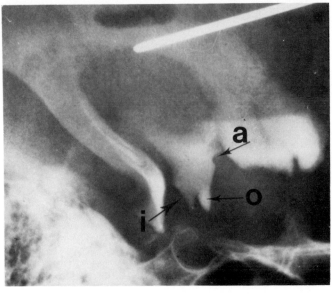

A

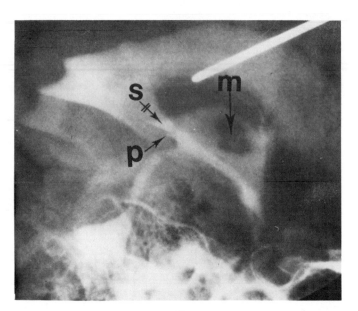

B

Figure 5.23. Radiological anatomy of the third ventricle. Conray ventriculogram performed in a patient with a small posterior fossa tumour and used here to illustrate the anatomy of the third ventricle. A. brow down and B. brow up radiographs. O = optic recess, i = infundibular recess, a = anterior commissure, m = massa intermedia, s = supra pineal recess, p = pineal recess.

increased osteoclastic activity on the inner wall of the sinus and osteoblastic activity on its outside. There is also a higher incidence of dural calcification in acromegaly. Fairly characteristic changes occurring in the mandible are: elongation of the ascending ramus, widening of the mandibular angle and protrusion of the occlusal surface of the mandible beyond the maxilla (prognathism). These deformities can be explained on the basis of overgrowth of that part of the mandible developed from Meckel's cartilage. Elongation of the mandible can be readily shown on the lateral skull radiograph by drawing a line along the lower margin of the horizontal ramus of the mandible and extending it backwards to the vertebral column. In normal adults, this line meets the disc between the 2nd and the 3rd vertebral bodies, whereas in acromegaly the line reaches a lower level (Trapnell and Bowerman, 1973).

The hand of the acromegalic patient is bulky and spade-shaped, mainly because of soft tissue hypertrophy. Radiologically the subcutaneous fat lines in the fingers disappear, there is enlargement of the tufts of the terminal phalanges, widening of the joint spaces and formation of bony excrescences at the insertion of ligaments and tendons. The latter occur practically anywhere in the skeleton. Similar changes take place in the feet, but the most striking feature is increased thickness of the heel pad, which, being related to the severity and the duration of the disease, enables sequential measurements to be used as an indication of the effect of therapy (Kho, Wright and Doyle, 1970).

From a neurological viewpoint, the changes occurring in the spine are of special interest (Chester and Chester, 1940). New bone formation may occur on the anterior surface of the vertebrae particularly in the thoracic region, but may be seen elsewhere in the spine. While new bone is formed anteriorly, bone resorption takes place posteriorly leading to abnormal scalloping (Figure 5.28). This may be due in part to thickening of the soft tissue contents within the spinal canal and is most obvious when it occurs in the lumbar region. It should not be misdiagnosed as being the result of an intraspinal tumour. However, we have seen a number of acromegalics who developed symptoms of lumbar canal stenosis and intermittent ischaemia of the cauda equina from excessive degeneration and new bone formation at the interarticular joints.

The Troell—Junet syndrome

This is a rare endocrinal complex consisting of acromegaly, toxic goitre (usually nodular), diabetes mellitus and hyperostosis of the skull vault. All reported cases were in females (Sherwood, 1953). Radiologically, patients suffering from these diseases cannot be differentiated from those having acromegaly alone, but thyroid swelling may be apparent on the chest radiograph.

The Sella in Cushing's Disease

In his classical paper on basophil adenoma of the pituitary gland Cushing (1932) wrote: 'A polyglandular syndrome hitherto supposed to be of cortico-adrenal origin characterised in its full-blown state by acute plethoric adiposity, by genital dystrophy, by osteoporosis, by vascular hypertension, and so on, has been found at autopsy in six out of eight instances to be associated with a pituitary adenoma. In all these cases the tumour was uniformly small in size measuring about 5 mm in diameter and only one out of twelve cases showed an abnormal pituitary fossa.' Cushing was of the opinion that the adrenal hyperplasia was secondary to a small basophil adenoma and questioned the accuracy of the histological examination when such a tumour was not found at autopsy.

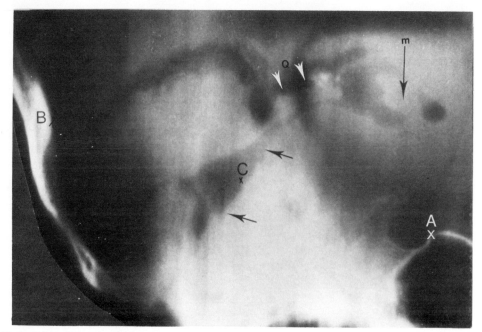

Figure 5.24A. Normal pneumoencephalogram. Twining's line. One of the most useful lines in assessing the position of the fourth ventricle in the sagittal plane is the Twining Line. This is a line drawn from the tuberculum sellae 'A' to the torcular Herophili 'B'. Normally the midpoint of Twining's line 'C' lies within the fourth ventricle, at or slightly posterior to its floor (horizontal black arrows). (m = mass intermedia, Q = quadrigeminal cistern or the cistern of great vein of Galen). Arrow heads point to the anterior cerebral artery.

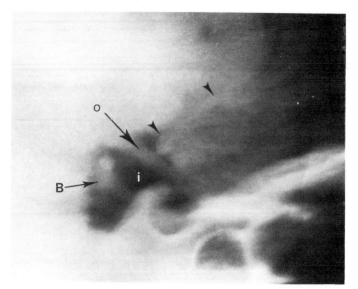

Figure 5.24B. Normal pneumoencephalogram. The subarachnoid cisterns around the sella. The pontine cistern lies between the ventral aspect of the pons and the clivus surrounding the basilar artery 'B'. It is continuous upwards with the interpeduncular cistern 'i'. The suprasellar cistern is a forward extension of the interpeduncular cistern from which it may be separated by a thin arachnoid membrane called Liliequist membrane (see Figure 5.24C). The suprasellar cistern is divided by the optic chiasm 'o' into two parts: one part lies above and in front of the chiasm (the prechiasmatic part or the cisterna chiasmatis) and the second lies below and posterior to the chiasm (postchiasmatic part).

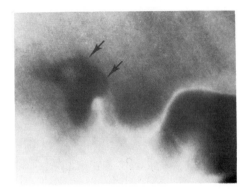

Figure 5.24C. Liliequist membrane (double arrows). This is a thin membrane lying in the subarachnoid space and it is generally considered to be the line of demarcation between the interpeduncular and the suprasellar cistern. Air is often held behind the Liliequist membrane on the initial radiographs but this should not be mistaken for the result of a suprasellar tumour. The membrane is straight or concave whereas the outline of a tumour is convex. Furthermore, the radiographs which are taken later during the procedure often demonstrate normal suprasellar cisterns. This is presumably due to rupture of the membrane under the force of air accumulating in the interpeduncular cistern.

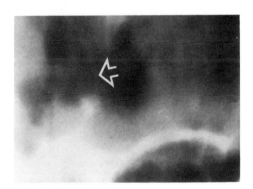

Figure 5.24D. In this case of wide subarachnoid spaces, Liliequist membrane is seen with unusual clarity.

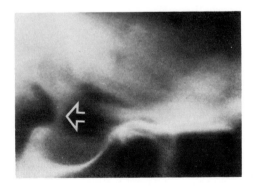

Figure 5.24E. The pituitary stalk (arrow) is well illustrated.

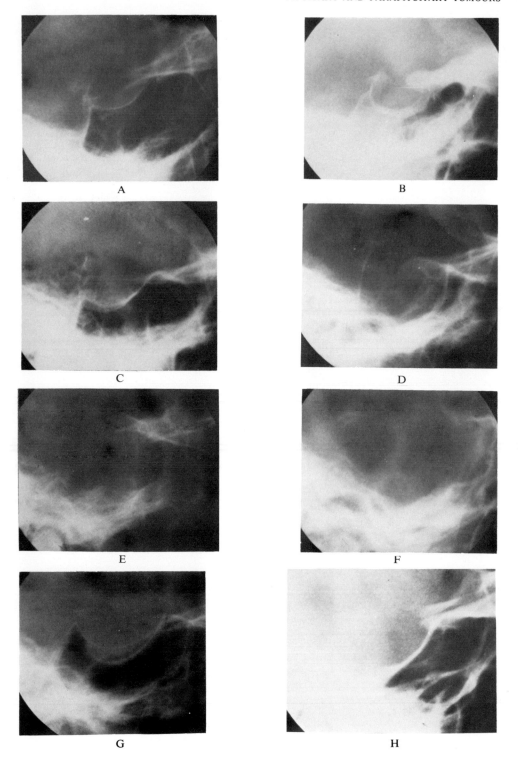

A

B

C

D

E

F

G

H

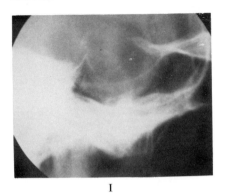

I

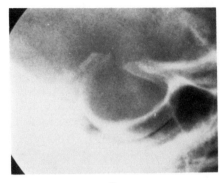

J

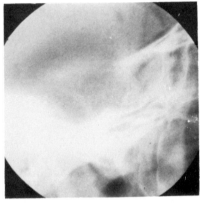

K

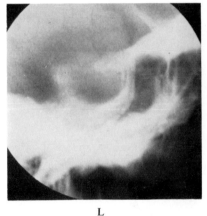

L

Figure 5.25. Sellar changes due to chromophobe adenoma. Note that in (A) the sella is normal in size but there is slight undermining of the anterior clinoids and thinning of the dorsum. In (B), the sellar area appears normal but the anterior wall of the floor is thin and excavated. In Figure (C) and (D) the dorsum sallae, being thin and stretched, indicates an intrasellar neoplasm. The posterior clinoids usually remain intact despite complete resorption of the dorsum as shown in Figures (E) and (F). That this observation is not infallible is shown in (G) and (H). In fact in (H) the posterior clinoids, the dorsum and part of the floor of the sella are completely wiped off which is far from being a feature of chromophobe adenoma, and in (G) it is mainly the sellar outlet which is enlarged. Figures (I) and (J) illustrate the classical pathological double outline of the sellar floor due to unilateral expansion of the tumour into the sphenoid sinus. Figure (K) shows complete destruction of the dorsum and sella which means that the tumour is invasive but it does not indicate that it is histologically malignant. Figure (L) shows some increased density of a non-pneumatised rim of cancellous bone around the sella, a feature which is often thought to be characteristic of craniopharyngioma, but here occurring in a chromophobe adenoma which is perhaps less invasive and slowly growing than in Figure (K).

Since that time other causes of Cushing's syndrome have been recognised, some iatrogenic and others occurring naturally. According to Rovit and Berry (1965), the majority of patients with the naturally occurring form of the disease have bilateral adrenal hyperplasia. About 15 to 20 per cent have adrenal adenomas or carcinomas capable of autonomous secretory activity. Macroscopic pituitary tumours are present in less than 10 per cent and occasionally the characteristic endocrinopathy is seen secondary to ectopic ACTH production in patients with malignant tumours of other organs, such as the lungs, pancreas, thymus and ovary. Knowlton (1953) studied the relation between pituitary and adrenal lesions in 98 autopsied cases of Cushing's disease and found that pituitary tumours of one sort or another were present in half the number of cases and basophilic adenoma occurred in one-third. It is extremely rare for the basophilic adenoma to give local symptoms or signs such as restriction of the visual fields or enlargement of the pituitary fossa. The pituitary–adrenal problem is further compounded by the fact that a number of pituitary tumours – mostly chromophobes – may manifest themselves clinically a few years after adrenalectomy (Rovit and Berry, 1965). Whether or not these tumours were present in a sub-clinical state prior to surgery is a matter of speculation. Furthermore, enlargement of the pituitary fossa may be seen in patients who have had bilateral adrenalectomy for Cushing's disease, but in whom the diagnosis of a pituitary lesion has never been established. Whether the sellar enlargement is due to hyperplasia of the pituitary gland or to an undiagnosed small intrasellar tumour is a difficult question to answer. Hyperpigmentation, increased plasma level of corticotrophins or restriction of the visual fields points to a pituitary origin and warrants thorough neuroradiological examination. A normal appearance of the sella on the plain skull radiographs does not exclude a suprasellar mass as shown in the case reported by Krieger, Krieger and Soffer (1964).

The extracranial skeletal abnormalities that may be associated with Cushing's syndrome are mainly due to generalised osteoporosis and diminished sensitivity to pain. Thus multiple vertebral collapse and rib fractures are common and may be asymptomatic. Callus formation is poor and areas of aseptic necrosis may be seen (Murray, 1960). In investigating patients with Cushing's syndrome, it should be remembered that in them purpura and a liability to bruising are common, thus they are liable to develop a large haematoma following angiography and it is preferable to avoid direct puncture of the cerebral vessels in these cases. The radiologist should also be aware of the fact that these patients may require steroid cover during the procedure, particularly if it is performed under general anaesthesia, and these investigations should not be undertaken without full liaison with the endocrinologist.

The sella in prolactin cell adenoma

It is well known that acromegaly may be associated with amenorrhoea and galactorrhoea, but perhaps less well known that a number of such patients, usually referred from infertility clinics, have no acromegalic features and in them estimation of growth hormone may be normal. This syndrome of amenorrhoea and galactorrhoea is often due to a prolactin-secreting pituitary microadenoma (Vezina and Sutton, 1974). Some of these patients may show an enlarged sella (Figure 5.29), but even in the absence of sellar enlargement, tomograms in the antero-posterior and lateral projections may reveal localised erosion or bulging which is otherwise difficult to detect. Prolactin cell adenomas are usually small in size, measuring five to seven mm in diameter and may be too small to produce any appreciable change in the sellar volume.

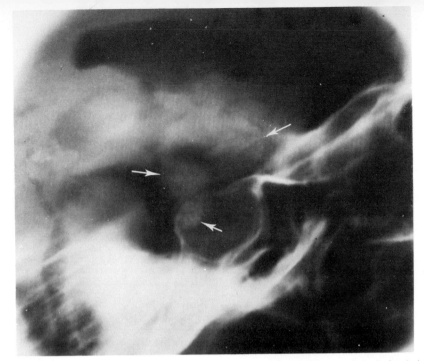

Figure 5.26. Nodular calcification in chromophobe adenoma. Pneumoencephalogram, lateral view in brow-up position: The suprasellar extension of the tumour is outlined by top arrows. Lower arrow points to the calcified part of the tumour.

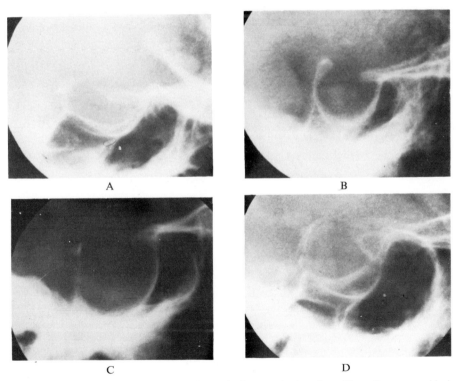

Figure 5.27. The sella in acromegaly. The main features in the above illustrations are: widening of the anteroposterior diameter in (a), deepening of the sella in (b), uniform expansion in (c) and double outline of the floor in (d).

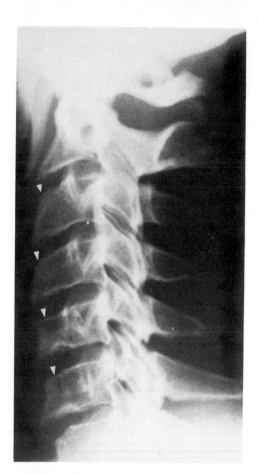 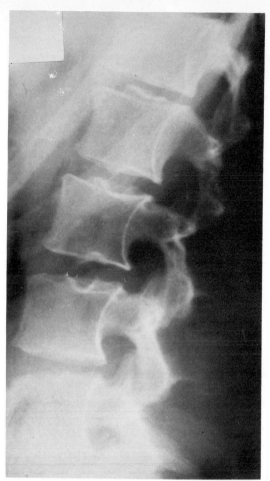

Figure 5.28. The spine in acromegaly. There is deposition of new bone on the anterior surface of the centrum as shown in the cervical region although it is more often seen in the thoracic spine. Scalloping of the posterior surface of the centrum is usually evident in the lumbar region.

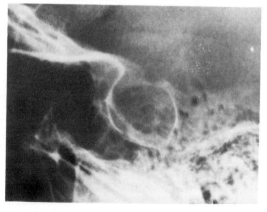

Figure 5.29. This sella belongs to a 38-year-old housewife with periodic mild galactorrhoea for about 16 years. She has four children, the youngest being 11 years. For about four years she has been on the contraceptive pill and since coming off it three years before this radiograph was taken, she has no menses.

Angiography in pituitary adenoma

The vascular displacement due to chromophobe adenoma and other pituitary tumours has been outlined previously (p. 115). On conventional angiography, pathological tumour circulation may appear in a small number of chromophobe adenomas (Figure 5.30). Using the magnification technique and subtraction, abnormal findings are detectable in a higher proportion of cases. These consist of enlargement of the meningo-hypophyseal trunk or abnormal vascularisation in the form of a 'blush'. So impressive are the results of magnification angiography in the diagnosis of pituitary tumours that it has been recommended as the examination of choice in preference to pneumoencephalography (Powell, Baker and Laws, 1974). These authors observed pathological changes in the meningo-hypophyseal trunk and abnormal tumour vascularity in all their cases.

Pneumoencephalography in pituitary adenoma

Pituitary adenomas produce two main abnormalities on the pneumoencephalogram, viz. elevation of the suprasellar cistern and deformation of the anterior recesses of the third ventricle (Figure 5.31). Air within the carotid cistern should not be mistaken for the suprasellar cistern (Figure 5.32). Where doubt exists autotomography, or preferably single cut tomography, is helpful (Lewtas and Jefferson, 1966). The presence of a visual field defect is usually indicative of suprasellar extension, so much so that in the past neurosurgeons were prepared to explore the chiasmal region even if such a lesion were not shown radiologically. With modern radiological equipment it is no longer difficult to demonstrate a small suprasellar extension or tumour recurrence.

Massive chromophobe adenomas are not uncommon. The tumour may extend downwards into the sphenoidal air sinus (Figure 5.33), upwards into the front lobes (Figure 5.34) or laterally beneath the temporal lobes (Figure 5.35). The majority of these large tumours are of the mixed variety and may lead to acromegalic features of varying severity.

RADIOLOGY OF CRANIOPHARYNGIOMA

Practically any type of sellar changes may be seen in cases of craniopharyngioma. Much depends on whether the site of origin of the tumour is above or below the diaphragma sellae (Figure 5.36). A tumour arising from the lower group of squamous epithelial islets tends to cause uniform expansion of the sella but, if the tumour arises from the upper group of cells, it causes widening of the sellar outlet. In suprasellar tumours there is no direct correlation between tumour size and the sellar changes, i.e. a large tumour growing in a cephalad direction may be present with little or no sellar change. There is a higher incidence of sellar change and tumour calcification in children than in adults (Figure 5.37). Table 5.1 is a comparative analysis of the radiographic findings in children and adults based on a retrospective study of 160 cases (Banna, 1973).

Calcification in craniopharyngioma does not differ in its morphological appearance from calcification occurring in any other tumour (Figure 5.38). It may be nodular, amorphous, fluffy or, very rarely, of the curvilinear, cystic type. It is usually in the mid-line but may occupy the outer part of the tumour only. Calcification may on rare occasions be within the sella or entirely behind the dorsum sellae.

At angiography there are no specific features which distinguish a craniopharyngioma from any other avascular suprasellar neoplasm. Among the 160 cases reviewed only one showed enlargement of the inferior hypophyseal artery, but vascular displacement of some

Table 5.1. Analysis of radiographic findings based on a retrospective study of 160 cases.

	Children (per cent)	Adults (per cent)
Tumour calcification	77.5	35
Sellar changes	70	50
They consist of:		
widened outlet	36	10
shortened dorsum	18	18
uniform expansion	13	17
destroyed	3	1
increased intracranial pressure	40	5
The skull radiographs were normal i.e. showing no sellar changes or tumour calcification	6	40

sort was noted in 74 per cent of children and 57 per cent of adults. When carotid angiography is performed, there are two observations which ought to be remembered. First, elevation of the anterior cerebral artery may not occur in the presence of an enormous tumour (Figure 5.39). In these cases, the tumour arises within the circle of Willis; it is often pear-shaped and the anterior cerebral arteries, related to the narrow part of the tumour, remain undisplaced. Second, some craniopharyngiomas grow primarily in a posterior direction, displacing the posterior part of the circle of Willis. In these cases vertebral angiography may be valuable (Figure 5.40).

As in other pituitary and parapituitary tumours pneumoencephalography gives a more satisfactory demonstration of the tumour size and extension (Figure 5.41). In cases of craniopharyngioma the effect of tumour growth on the suprasellar cistern varies. If the tumour arises from the upper group of cells and is predominantly suprasellar, the cistern is usually completely obliterated. On the other hand a tumour arising from within the sella tends first to displace the sub-arachnoid space (Figure 5.42). We have not seen a suprasellar cistern displaced downwards by a suprasellar craniopharyngioma. The latter obliterates the cistern at an earlier stage than those arising within the sella itself.

Ventricular dilatation is common in craniopharyngioma and was noted in 74 per cent of children and 45 per cent of adults, an incidence which is much higher than in chromophobe adenoma. This is due to the invasive nature of the craniopharyngioma compared to the benign extracerebral location of pituitary adenomas. Obstruction of the ventricular system is usually due to occlusion of the foramen of Monro, but there are cases in which the tumour growth encroaches on the aqueduct or displaces the fourth ventricle. In these the pontine cistern will be also posteriorly displaced in keeping with the extra-neuronal origin of the tumour (Figure 5.43).

Another contrast study which may be required to outline the cystic component of the tumour is cystography. Air or a sterile barium suspension (Steripaque) is injected into the cyst and appropriate radiographs in the brow-up and brow-down positions are taken. Barium adheres to the tumour capsule and 1 to 3 cm are usually sufficient to show its entire surface. This may be helpful to assess the size of the lesion following treatment.

RADIOLOGY OF SUPRASELLAR MENINGIOMA

Meningiomas occurring in relation to the hypophysis may be suprasellar, parasellar or intrasellar. The first arise from the tuberculum sellae, the diaphragma sellae or the planum

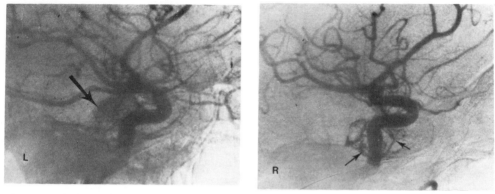

Figure 5.30. Right and left conventional carotid angiogram of a very vascular chromophobe adenoma. Arrows point to abnormal vessels and tumour circulation.

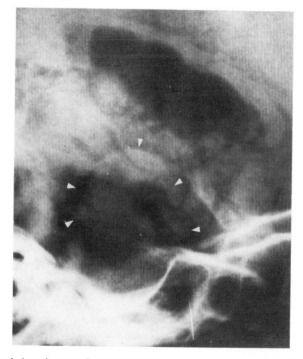

Figure 5.31. Chromophobe adenoma. Pneumoencephalogram: Lateral view in the brow-up position. The tumour is separated from the surrounding brain by a line of cleavage which *occasionally* fills with air and outlining its whole circumference (arrows).

sphenoidale; the second from the inner third of the sphenoidal ridge or the greater wing of the sphenoid bone. In the third and rarest location the tumour arises from that part of the arachnoid membrane which may herniate below the diaphragma sellae through a wide orifice for the pituitary stalk. Tumours in any of these locations are much more common in females.

The bony changes that may occur in association with suprasellar meningioma are shown in Figure 5.44, but the most important characteristic change is hyperostosis. The overall incidence of hyperostosis in meningioma is about 23 per cent, but it varies according to the tumour site, being highest in tuberculum sellae meningioma (Traub, 1961). In a series of 45 cases, di Chiro and Lindgren (1952) found hyperostosis in no less than 50 per cent. The newly formed bone often involves the planum sphenoidale, but may extend laterally to the anterior clinoids and the optic foramina or posteriorly into the floor of the sella. It may be dense or mound-like in one case and relatively thin in another. The surface of the newly formed bone is usually irregular and never as sharply defined as the normal cortical bone.

A comparatively low incidence of sellar changes occurs in cases of suprasellar meningioma. di Chiro and Lindgren found definite sellar changes in the form of enlargement with destruction of the floor or the dorsum in 20 per cent of cases. In 55 per cent the sella was normal and in the remaining 25 per cent no definite changes were found although the dorsum was sometimes short. The incidence of calcification in suprasellar meningioma is also small, being approximately 6 per cent, compared to 10 per cent which is the overall incidence of calcification in meningioma.

At angiography, enlargement of the hypophyseal arteries (Figure 5.45) and tumour 'blush' (Figure 5.46) were observed in about one-third of our cases, but a higher incidence may be shown by magnification angiography. Occasionally meningiomas close to the internal carotid artery or the optic nerve encircle these structures and in such cases total excision of the tumour is practically impossible (Figure 5.47).

At pneumoencephalography, a filling defect in the anterior part of the third ventricle caused by meningioma is indistinguishable from that caused by other tumours. One distinguishing feature of meningioma, however, may be noted if the air in the subarachnoid space surrounds the tumour (Figure 5.48).

OPTIC NERVE GLIOMA

The clinical manifestations of optic chiasm glioma have been discussed in Chapter 2. The skull radiographs in these cases may show enlargement of the optic foramen, alteration in the sella, manifestations of raised intracranial pressure, or they may be entirely normal (Holman, 1959). The x-ray projection which is commonly used to outline the optic foramen is the Rhese–Goalwin projection, in which the optic foramen is projected within the infero-lateral quadrant of the orbit (Farberov, 1937). Using standard radiographic techniques, the average maximum diameter of the canal is 4.0 mm in the newborn, increasing to 5.0 mm when the child is about 6 months of age and reaching the adult size of 5.5 mm at about 5 years (Evans, Schwartz and Chutorian, 1963). Both optic canals are usually symmetrical, varying less than 1.0 mm in 98 per cent of normal skulls. Taveras and Wood (1964) consider an optic foramen to be enlarged if its diameter exceeds 6.5 mm or if there is a difference of 2.0 mm or more between both sides. On a technically satisfactory radiograph, the optic canal appears almost circular or slightly elliptical in shape, but slight difference in the angulation of the longitudinal axis of the canal may cause some asymmetry. A rare, but important anatomical variation in the shape of the optic canal results from alteration in the course of the ophthalmic artery. Normally, the artery

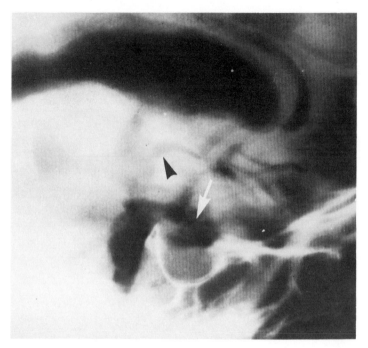

Figure 5.32. Chromophobe adenoma. Pneumoencephalogram: Lateral view in brow-up position. The carotid cistern (white arrow) should not be mistaken for the suprasellar cistern. The tumour extends further upwards into the third ventricle (black arrow).

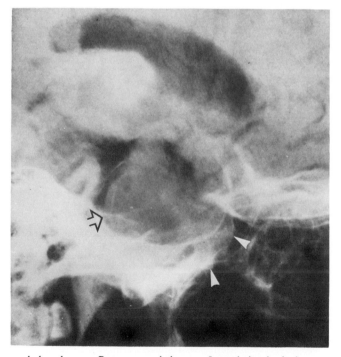

Figure 5.33. Chromophobe adenoma. Pneumoencephalogram: Lateral view in the brow-up position. There is massive extension of the tumour into the sphenoidal air sinus and nasopharynx (arrows).

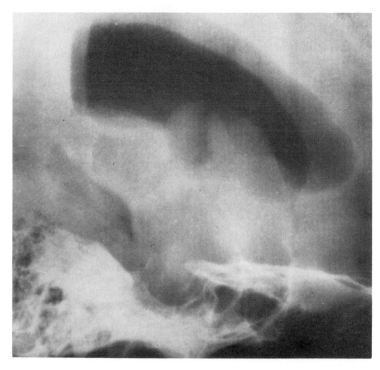

Figure 5.34. Chromophobe adenoma. Pneumoencephalogram: Lateral radiograph in the brow-up position. There is massive extension of the tumour in a frontal direction and relatively slight intrasellar expansion.

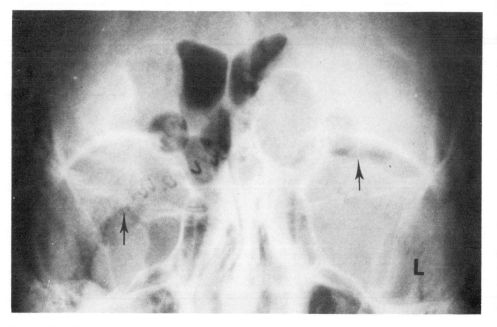

Figure 5.35. Chromophobe adenoma with subtemporal extension. Pneumoencephalogram: antero-posterior radiograph. Vertical arrows point to the temporal horns.

enters the orbital cavity through the optic canal, below and lateral to the nerve. Occasionally, it may lie within a groove or a tunnel, usually limited to the cranial end of the canal and the anomaly may be unilateral or bilateral. The presence of a notch in the inferior part of the canal should not therefore be considered as pathological.

Primary neoplasm of the optic nerve is the most frequent cause of widening of the optic canal. A widened optic foramen is also the most specific radiological feature of optic nerve glioma (Figure 5.49). Evans, Schwartz and Chutorian (1963) found an abnormally enlarged optic foramen in 83 per cent of the children with glioma of one optic nerve and 67 per cent of those with glioma of the chiasma. In spite of the enlargement, the canal retains its distinct regular cortical margins. This is probably because the growing bone of the child moulds itself around the slowly growing tumour. Bone erosion is more liable to occur if the tumour enlarges rapidly within a fixed canal of an adult. Attention should be drawn to widening or erosion which may be limited to the cranial or orbital meatus of the canal and is difficult to see on the Rhese–Goalwin projection but may be easier to detect on lateral or basal tomography of the skull.

Enlargement of the optic foramen may be seen in cases of neurofibromatosis due to generalised hypertrophy of the connective tissue and as part of the orbital manifestations of the disease. These include: generalised orbital enlargement, widening of the superior orbital fissure, bony defects in the orbital wall, elevation of the lesser wing of the sphenoid bone and deformation of the sella turcica (Burrows, 1963). Even in the presence of these abnormalities, it is difficult to exclude the possibility of glioma unless vision is intact. Other causes of optic canal enlargement arc rarc and include meningioma, retinoblastoma, choroid carcinoma, ophthalmic artery aneurysm or arteriovenous malformation and chronic raised intracranial pressure (Potter and Trokel, 1971). Bilateral enlargement of the optic canals have been shown also in association with craniopharyngioma (Block, Gore and Jimenez, 1973).

The sellar changes which are suggestive of, but not limited to, optic chiasm glioma result from deepening and excavation of the sulcus interopticus, often described as the J-shaped sella. Tumour calcification is rare, but in some series nodular calcified foci were seen in 20 per cent of the cases (Schuster and Westberg, 1967). At pneumoencephalography, the presence of a filling defect in the anterior portion of the third ventricle is, by itself, indistinguishable from that seen in any other tumour (Figure 5.50). Nevertheless, a definitive diagnosis may be possible if the deformity is interpreted in the light of other manifestations of the disease as shown in Figure 5.51; or in the presence of a wide chiasmatic insertion due to splaying of the optic and infundibular recesses by the thickened chiasm (Schuster and Westberg, 1967); also if the optic nerve within the suprasellar cistern is seen to be abnormally thickened (Evans et al, 1963).

Other gliomas occurring in the suprasellar region may arise primarily in the floor of the third ventricle. This may be seen in patients with manifestations of hypothalamic dysfunction or in infants with the diencephalic syndrome. Tumour calcification may occur in a small number of these tumours, rendering their differentiations from other lesions in the sellar area much more difficult (Figure 5.10).

INTRACRANIAL CHORDOMA

It is important to include the clinical manifestations of intracranial chordoma in the radiology section since it is not a primary pituitary lesion and may require, in addition to the routine skull radiographs, special views of the area related to the patient's symptomatology. These may include tomograms of the clivus, the retropharyngeal space,

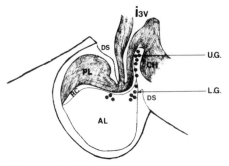

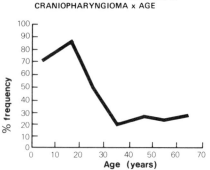

FREQUENCY OF CALCIFICATION IN
CRANIOPHARYNGIOMA x AGE

Figure 5.36. Diagrammatic illustrations of squamous epithelial islets. Squamous epithelial cells that are remnants of the cranio-pharyngeal duct are present in clusters or 'islets', shown as solid black dots in the diagram. They occur in varying size, number and distribution in a large proportion of nor-mal individuals but in some, it is believed, they may give rise to craniopharyngioma. There are mainly two groups of epithelial islets; an upper (UG) lying along the anterior surface of

Figure 5.37. Frequency of calcification in craniopharyngioma x age.

the pituitary infundibulum and a lower (LG) lying beneath the diaphragma sellae. (AL = anterior lobe, PL = posterior lobe, RC =Rathke's cleft, DS = diaphragma sellae, CH = optic chiasm, i3V = infundibular recess of third ventricle.)

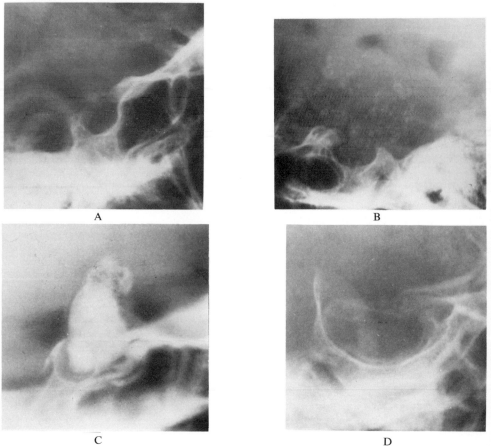

Figure 5.38. Types of calcification in craniopharyngioma. A. nodular, B. granular or punctate, C. amorphous or homogeneous, D. curvilinear.

the orbital fissures, the petrous apices or the entire skull base in the submento-vertical projection.

The most common symptoms of clivus chordoma are headache, visual disturbances, nasal obstruction (from ventral extension of the tumour into the nasopharynx) and pain in the neck (Givner, 1945). Diplopia due to paralysis of the lateral rectus muscle, less frequently of the medial rectus, occurs in about one-third of the cases. Visual field defects, optic atrophy or papilloedema due to compression of the optic chiasm are also common. Although the tumour is typically a mid-line lesion, there is a pronounced tendency for involvement of the cranial nerves to be unilateral and even if the involvement is bilateral, it is more complete or widespread on one side than the other. The visual field defects are similar to those caused by other lesions in the sellar region, but in chordoma functional disturbance of the hypophysis is rare and occurs later in the course of the disease. Headache usually precedes the changes in visual fields which is reversed in pituitary tumours.

In addition to the abducent, the trochlear, the oculomotor and the optic nerves, practically any cranial nerve may be involved. Chordoma may present as a cerebello-pontine angle tumour affecting primarily the acoustic, the vestibular and the facial nerves. It may present as a lesion in the region of the jugular fossa involving the glossopharyngeal, vagus and accessory nerves and further extension may involve the hypoglossal canal and the foramen magnum, the latter resulting in neck stiffness and pain accentuated by head movements.

Second in frequency to cranial nerve palsies are the symptoms and signs resulting from compression and displacement of the pons, medulla or upper part of the cervical cord. They include long tract sensory and motor disturbances in addition to involvement of cranial nerve nuclei.

The radiological findings in cases of intracranial chordoma include bone destruction, soft tissue swelling and tumour calcification (Schechter, Liebeskind and Azar-Kia, 1974). Bone destruction occurs in approximately 85 per cent of cases. It is entirely osteolytic without any reaction in the form of periosteal new bone formation or osteosclerosis (Figure 5.52) and usually involves the spheno-occipital synchondrosis, which is the commonest site of origin of these tumours. The lesion may then extend into the clivus, the base of the dorsum sellae, the sphenoid sinus or the apices of the petrous bones. Larger tumours may creep anteriorly along the skull base causing destruction of the optic foramen, the orbital fissure and the ethmoidal sinus. They may grow laterally beneath the temporal lobe causing destruction of the greater wing of the sphenoid or into the cerebello-pontine angle and the jugular foramen. The sella is involved in approximately two-thirds of the cases but, unlike the appearances in pituitary tumours, it is never ballooned and undermining of the anterior clinoids occurs only in massive lesions. The base of the dorsum sellae is affected first and later the destructive process may extend into the posterior clinoids and into other parts of the sella.

A retropharyngeal soft tissue mass may be present in about one-third of the cases, but it may be shown only on lateral tomograms of the nasopharynx or the skull base. Differentiation from carcinoma of the sphenoid sinus or the nasopharynx may be difficult.

Tumour calcification in chordoma was thought to be rare, but a recent review study of a large number of cases indicated that calcium deposits of some sort may be seen in approximately 50 per cent of cases (Schechter et al, 1974). These authors stated that calcification was in fact a feature of chordoma. This may be reticular-like fine lacework, solid and nodular, scattered in flecks, 'cystic' or mixed. In the presence of minute flecks of calcium it is often difficult to distinguish between sequestrated bone and tumour calcification. Similarly a calcified chordoma (Figure 5.53) may be difficult to differentiate from cartilaginous tumours in the skull base (Minagi and Newton, 1969).

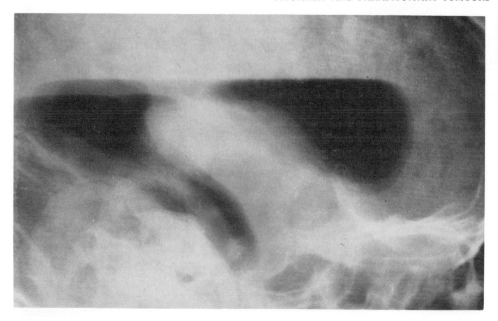

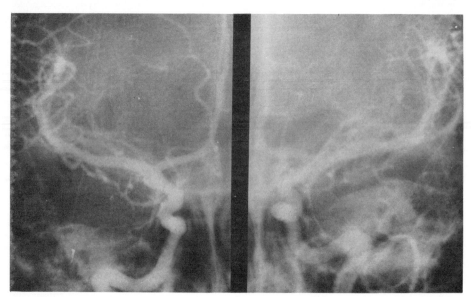

Figure 5.39. Bilateral carotid angiogram and ventriculogram of the same patient. A large craniopharyngioma causing obstruction of the interventricular foramen, yet no elevation of the horizontal portion of the anterior cerebral arteries. In such a case the tumour grows within the circle of Willis behind the anterior cerebral arteries.

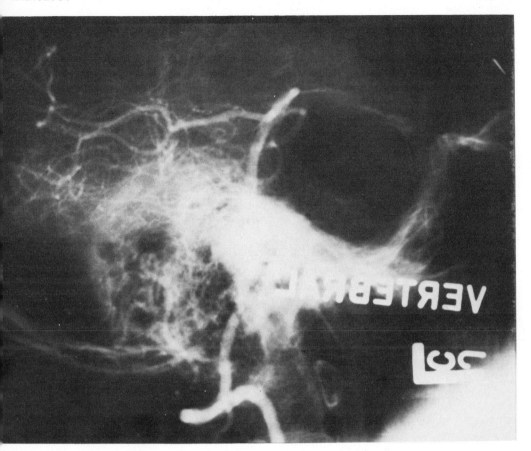

Figure 5.40. Vertebral angiogram. The basilar artery is posteriorly displaced by a craniopharyngioma extending in a retrosellar direction behind the clivus.

At angiography the most important changes are seen in relation to the basilar artery which is invariably posteriorly displaced (Figure 5.54). The artery may also be deviated across the mid-line if the tumour growth is eccentric. Chordomas are avascular tumours and can be easily differentiated from a clivus meningioma by their avascularity. The second most helpful observation at angiography is deformation of the cavernous portion of the internal carotid artery. This may be displaced forward and laterally by the intrasphenoid part of the tumour, as may also occur with large pituitary adenomas. There are numerous other types of vascular displacements which may be seen in association with chordoma depending on the size and extension of the tumour.

At pneumoencephalography attempts should be made to outline the pontine cistern. This can be achieved simply by extending the head during air introduction. The main finding in cases of clivus chordoma is posterior displacement of the pontine cistern and the fourth ventricle. The former indicates that the lesion is extraneuronal and rules out the possibility of pontine glioma which also displaces the fourth ventricle posteriorly. If the cistern fails to fill at air-study, a vertebral angiogram should be performed to show that the basilar artery and the anterior ponto-mesencephalic vein are posteriorly displaced. The extension of the tumour along the skull base may also be outlined at pneumoencephalography (Figure 5.54B). A moderate degree of ventricular dilatation may

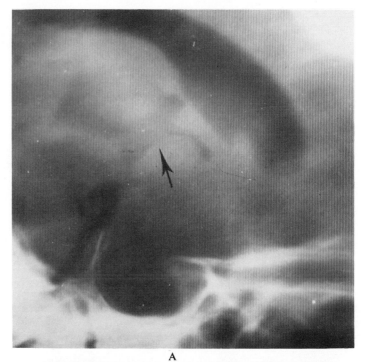

A

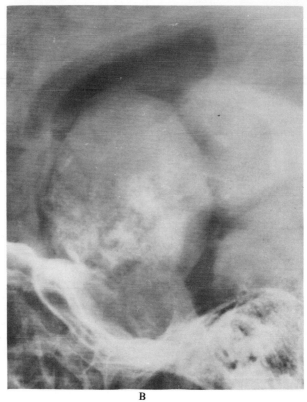

B

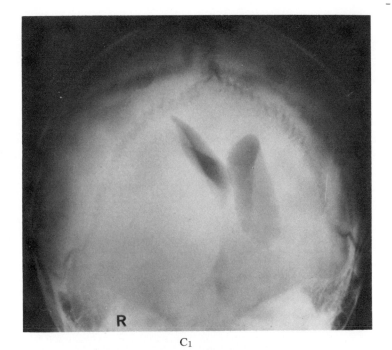

C_1

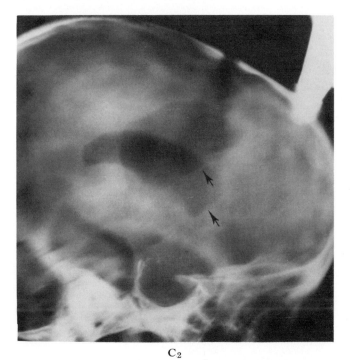

C_2

Figure 5.41. Craniopharyngioma: tumour size and extension. A. filling defect in the anterior part of the third ventricle. B. Encroachment on the foramen of Monro and the floor of the lateral ventricles. C_1 and C_2: Tumour extension into the frontal lobes.

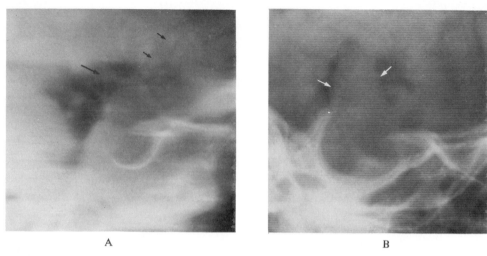

A   B

Figure 5.42. Intrasellar craniopharyngioma with suprasellar extension. The outline of the tumour is shown by air in the basal cisterns. Note the relationship of the tumour to neighbouring structures in Figure A. Long arrow points to the optic nerve and short arrows to the subarachnoid space around the anterior cerebral artery.

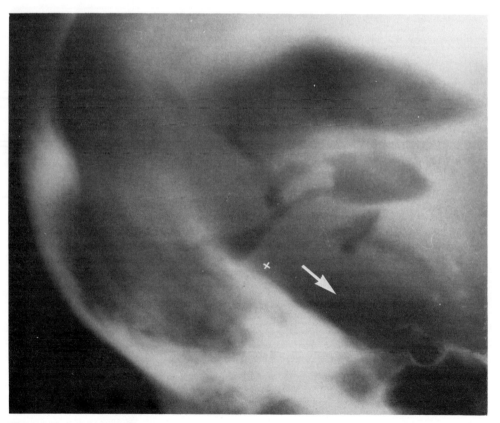

Figure 5.43. Craniopharyngioma: tumour growth into the posterior fossa. The pontine cistern (arrow) and the fourth ventricle are posteriorly displaced. The Twining point (cross) lies in front of the fourth ventricle.

result from encroachment on the interventricular foramen or the aqueduct, but this occurs only in massive lesions and at a later stage of the disease. Patients do not often survive to develop a marked degree of hydrocephalus.

Management of Chordoma

Because of the location of the tumour and its invasion of the skull base, total surgical removal is impossible. Surgery is, however, indicated in order to confirm the diagnosis, and to decompress the optic nerves and chiasm. Following partial removal of the tumour, x-ray therapy is usually given. According to Dahlin and MacCarty (1952), radiation therapy does not seem to alter the course of the disease appreciably, although earlier Wood and Himadi (1950) stated that irradiation has a beneficial effect in some cases. Following irradiation bone regeneration may occur (Figure 5.52), but recurrence is common and the lesion is usually fatal within five to ten years. Only a very small proportion of patients having spheno-occipital chordoma survive longer than 15 years.

CHOLESTEATOMA

As stated in the pathology section, suprasellar dermoid and epidermoid cysts (cholesteatoma) are encapsulated extracerebral tumours to be included in the differential diagnosis of suprasellar masses, particularly in adults in the absence of endocrinal abnormality. The skull radiographs may show curvilinear calcification, the brain scintigram is normal and at pneumoencephalography the tumour, which is avascular at angiography, may be separated from the surrounding brain by a thin layer of air in the sub-arachnoid spaces.

SUPRASELLAR GERMINOMA

This exceedingly rare tumour has no specific radiological features, but it should be considered in the differential diagnosis of invasive tumours in the suprasellar area. More so, if the patient is a young male adult having diabetes insipidus at the time of initial presentation, or occurring suddenly in response to corticosteroids. In this context, attention should be drawn to the fact that diabetes insipidus is induced when the neurohypophysis and the hypothalamus are affected without interruption of the function of the adenohypophysis. Symptoms of diabetes insipidus may begin to disappear if the function of the adenohypophysis is involved. Similarly, if the function of the adenohypophysis and neurohypophysis are affected from the beginning, diabetes insipidus may not be apparent clinically, but even in such cases, it is unveiled upon administration of steroids (Kageyama, 1971).

Radiologically, tumour calcification is rare in germinoma and only a few cases are associated with abnormal pituitary fossa. It has been estimated that sellar changes occur in approximately 20 per cent of the cases. The tumour usually arises above the sella and at pneumoencephalography, is associated with a filling defect in the anterior portion of the third ventricle and obliteration of the suprasellar cistern. Only in advanced cases does the tumour extend into the confines of the sella. An exceptionally rare, or perhaps unique, case was seen by the author in which the main tumour mass was within the sella and was outlined by air in the suprasellar cistern, in a fashion similar to chromophobe adenoma. This was a 15 year old boy with headaches, bitemporal hemianopia and hypopituitarism.

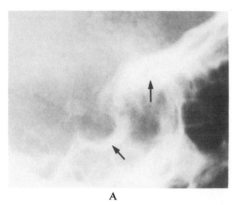

A

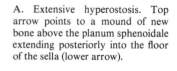

Figure 5.44. Sellar changes in suprasellar and parasellar meningioma.

A. Extensive hyperostosis. Top arrow points to a mound of new bone above the planum sphenoidale extending posteriorly into the floor of the sella (lower arrow).

B. The dorsum sellae and the floor of the sella are destroyed. There is excessive sclerosis of the partially pneumatised sphenoidal sinus.

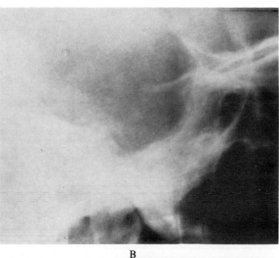

B

C. Absorption of the lamina dura of the sella and dorsum sellae similar to that resulting from raised intracranial pressure or pituitary adenoma.

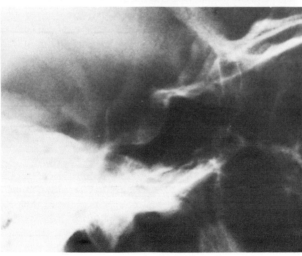

C

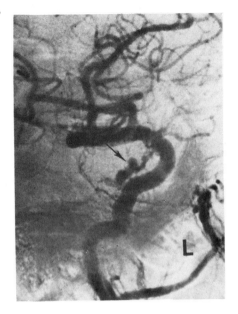 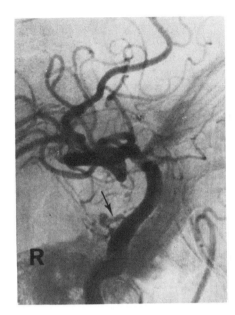

Figure 5.45. Meningioma. Right side: The cavernous part of the internal carotid artery is deformed and its intracranial part is elevated. Arrow points to the meningo-hypophyseal artery. Left side: Arrow points to an enormous superior hypophyseal artery. This was a large tumour extending in a parasellar and suprasellar direction.

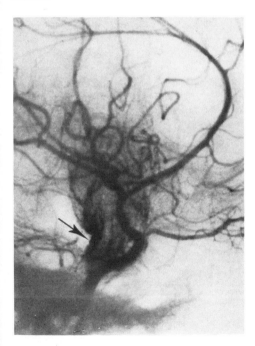 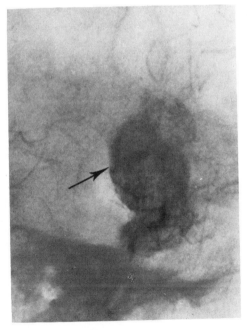

Figure 5.46. Meningioma. Early and late phase of carotid angiogram showing classical meningioma 'blush'. In this case the tumour probably arose from the diaphragma sellae. At operation, the tumour was fixed to the optic nerves and chiasm and could not be removed. (By courtesy of Dr. W. H. P. Shepherd.)

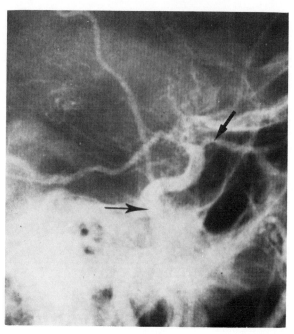

Figure 5.47. Parasellar meningioma. In this case the tumour has encircled the internal carotid artery (lower arrow) resulting in complete occlusion beyond the origin of the ophthalmic (top arrow) and posterior cerebral arteries. Small tumour vessels from the carotid siphon can be seen. (By courtesy of the editor of *Clinical Radiology*.)

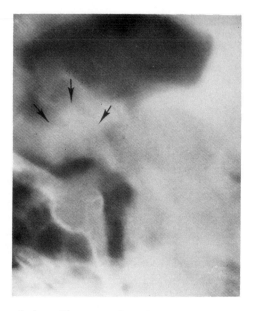

Figure 5.48. Suprasellar meningioma. The tumour circumference in this case was outlined by air (arrows).

Diabetes insipidus was absent at the time of clinical presentation, but became evident following the administration of corticosteroids in preparation for surgery – an event which is probably unknown in adenoma and is rare in other tumours. It should draw attention to involvement of the neurohypophyseal tract which is more common in germinoma (Banna et al, 1976).

MASSIVE BERRY ANEURYSM

Aneurysms large enough to distort the ventricular system are uncommon. They can present a difficult diagnostic problem and the pathological nature of the disease is sometimes not thought of, even after the most careful and exhaustive clinical examination. However, to the surgeon who has undertaken the removal of a suprasellar tumour only to discover at operation that it is an aneurysm, this type of lesion is an ever present possibility. No surgeon would wish to explore the case shown in Figure 5.55 without knowing its nature.

The difficulty in diagnosis of large aneurysms is due to the fact that not many bleed into the subarachnoid space. They have thick walls consisting of massive mural thrombus, and their symptoms are due to their space occupying effect. Bull (1969) emphasised the variability in the mode of clinical presentation of these aneurysms and stated that many present with visual symptoms which may be associated with headache, and on examination visual field defects may be found. Among other authors, Bird et al (1970) stressed again the point that unruptured aneurysms of the supraclinoid portion of the internal carotid artery may present with progressive visual failure, and are impossible to differentiate, prior to angiography, from other suprasellar tumours.

As important as the visual symptoms, or perhaps even more so but less well known, are mental changes that may be associated with massive lesions at the base of the brain. In Bull's series of 22 patients with massive aneurysms dementia was a main clinical manifestation in six who had been subjected to pneumoencephalography in order to confirm or refute the presence of cerebral atrophy.

ARACHNOID CYSTS

Arachnoid cysts in the region of the sella turcica are rare but should be included in the differential diagnosis of space occupying lesions within or above the sella (Banna, 1974). Before considering the various types, it is important that one should be familiar with the normal anatomy of the meninges in relation to the sella.

The Normal Anatomy of the Meninges in Relation to the Hypophysis Cerebri

According to Wislocki (1937) the epithelial hypophysis in man loses its connection with the oral cavity and comes to lie in the diffuse mesenchyme at the base of the brain before the meninges in this region are differentiated. As the dura mater develops and forms the diaphragma sellae, it prevents the development of the pia-arachnoid membrane around the body of the pituitary gland. Thus, between the glandular element of the pituitary gland and the sphenoidal air sinus, there are three structures: the capsule of the gland, a fibro-vascular layer of connective tissue and the floor of the sella. No subarachnoid space is present. Although the pituitary gland is not invested by the meninges, the pia-arachnoid does not terminate above the sella by forming a collar around the stalk. Instead, it provides

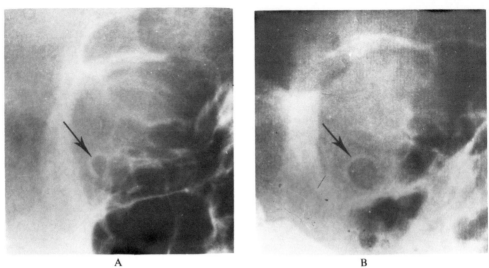

A   B

Figure 5.49. Optic nerve glioma. A. Normal optic foramen (Rhese position). B. Enlargement due to glioma of the optic nerve.

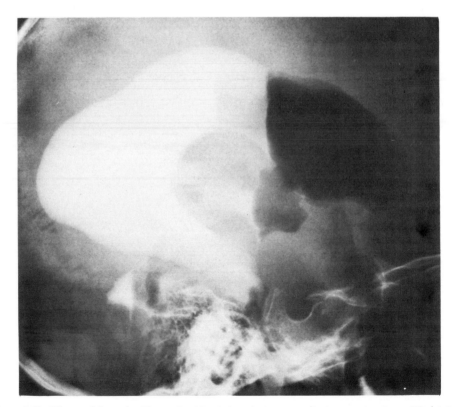

Figure 5.50. Glioma of the optic chiasm. Combined air and conray ventriculogram showing a filling defect in the anterior portion of the third ventricle which is indistinguishable from that caused by craniopharyngioma.

a loose covering that extends through the opening in the diaphragma sellae. If the infundibular foramen is large, it allows the sub-arachnoid space to come into contact with the hypophysis cerebri, and in these cases a large suprasellar cistern extending into the confines of the sella may be seen at pneumoencephalography. There are three types of arachnoid 'cysts' which may be seen in the sellar region (Figure 5.56):

Non-Communicating Cysts

These are not in continuity with the basal cisterns. The clinical picture and the radiological appearances of this type of lesion are indistinguishable from any non-calcified suprasellar neoplasm (Figure 5.57).

Communicating Cysts

Unlike the preceding type, cysts communicating with the sub-arachnoid space can be shown by pneumoencephalography (Figure 5.58). They are less likely to produce symptoms because of their free communication with the sub-arachnoid space, but the cyst may be large enough to obstruct the interventricular foramen (Sansregret et al, 1969).

Intrasellar Arachnoid Cysts

This is an extension of the suprasellar cistern into the pituitary fossa, i.e. it is a pouch or a diverticulum rather than a cyst. Its communication with the cistern may be wide or narrow depending on the size of its orifice. At pneumoencephalography, air may be retained within the diverticulum, which then appears as an intrasellar cyst (Figure 5.59). This appearance has received more attention in the recent literature under the heading 'empty' sella syndrome (Kaufman, 1968; Lee and Adams, 1968) an entity which needs some clarification and will, therefore, be separately considered.

'Empty' Sella Syndrome

Analysing the various causes of non-traumatic cerebrospinal fluid rhinorrhoea, Ommaya et al (1968) discovered that two out of eight patients had enlargement of the pituitary fossa associated with thinning and atrophy of the floor of the sella. At pneumoencephalography, the sella in these two patients was largely occupied by hernia of the arachnoid membrane and was thus described as 'empty' sella. Unfortunately, ever since that term was introduced, it has been used indiscriminately to describe practically any pituitary fossa which at pneumoencephalography shows some air beneath the assumed position of the diaphragma sellae. It should be clearly understood that herniation of the arachnoid membrane through a wide infundibular foramen with or without enlargement of the pituitary fossa is frequently seen in normal healthy individuals and in them it has no clinical significance (El-Gammal and Allen Jr, 1972; Kaufman and Chamberlin Jr, 1972). The herniated pouch may enlarge in the presence of raised intracranial pressure from any cause, including benign intracranial hypertension (Weisberg, Housepian and Saur, 1975) and the Pickwickian syndrome. The enlargement occurs under the effect of increased CSF pressure wave and may lead to erosion and enlargement of the pituitary fossa analogous to the creation of vault excavations by the arachnoid granulations (Ommaya et al, 1968). The

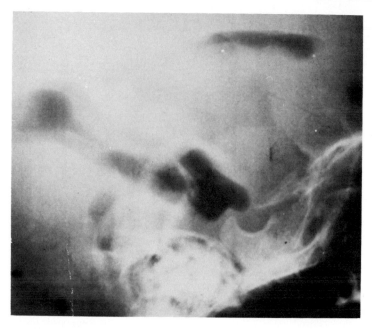

Figure 5.51. Optic chiasm glioma. In this case a definitive pathological diagnosis of the suprasellar tumour was possible because (a) The child was less than one year of age (uncommon age group for craniopharyngioma) (b) Loss of vision was an early sign (c) The J-shaped sella.

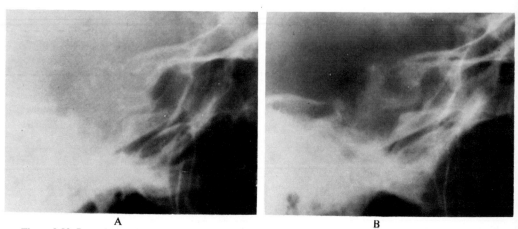

A   B

Figure 5.52. Bone destruction in chordoma. A. There is evidence of bone destruction in the clivus and dorsum sellae and small sequestrated bony fragments can be seen. B. Two years after irradiation: some bone regeneration is seen.

arachnoid membrane may also descend into the sella following surgery, irradiation or spontaneous infarction of pituitary adenoma; this type of case is sometimes referred to as secondary 'empty' sella syndrome (See page 22). Occasionally, a sella is described as 'empty' when its cavity is largely occupied by ballooned recesses of the third ventricle. This is more liable to occur in cases of chronic hydrocephalus, often due to aqueduct stenosis (Figure 5.14) and sometimes associated with mild hypopituitarism (Coenegracht et al, 1975). The primary 'empty' sella, being a frequent finding, may therefore be seen in association with many disease states, including endocrinopathies. It has not, to my knowledge, been established as a cause of Forbes-Albright syndrome. There are, however, very few cases, usually women in menopausal age, in whom the empty sella may be a cause of headache and visual deterioration. This has been attributed to the following effects of the herniated arachnoid pouch (Mortara and Norrell, 1970):
1. Thinning of the optic chiasm from the continuous transmitted pulsations of CSF.
2. Kinking of the optic nerve or chiasm.
3. Downward pressure on the anterior cerebral arteries by the dilated third ventricle, compressing the optic nerves or chiasm.

In conclusion, therefore, the presence of intrasellar arachnoid 'cysts', pouches or diverticulae is often referred to as 'empty' sella syndrome or primary 'empty' sella syndrome. In the majority of cases, this finding has no pathological significance, but there are a few cases in which thinning of the sellar floor may lead to the escape of CSF into the sphenoid sinus or to headache and visual impairment. It is probable that the condition in these patients is of different aetiology. Because it is more common in menopausal women, it has been suggested that it could have resulted from partial infarction of the pituitary gland, or from the return of the gland to its normal size following its enlargement during pregnancy. It has also been suggested that herniation of the arachnoid membrane might have occurred subsequent upon infarction of a small symptomless chromophobe adenoma which existed beforehand and caused some enlargement or erosion of the pituitary fossa (Brisman, Hughes and Mount, 1969).

SELLA CHANGES DUE TO EXTRACRANIAL DISEASES

Malignant Tumours of the nasopharynx

Carcinoma of the nasopharynx is common among the inhabitants of the Southeast Provinces of China, where it is the most frequent cancer in men and the third most frequent in women after cancer of the uterine cervix and of the breast (Chiang and Griem, 1973). The reason for this prevalence is not known but genetic and environmental factors have been suggested. In the white population carcinoma of the nasopharynx is rare and as a possible cause of cranial nerve palsy it may be overlooked. The tumour usually begins in the pharyngeal recess (Rosenmüller's fossa) close to the foramen lacerum, the most commonly involved part of the skull base. Lying immediately above the foramen lacerum is the cavernous sinus containing the third, fourth, fifth and sixth cranial nerves which are therefore liable to disturbance by the tumour. Of these the sixth nerve is the one lying lowest in the cavernous sinus closest to the sagittal plane and is usually the first cranial nerve to be affected. Thus double vision is one of the earliest symptoms and may progress to total ophthalmoplegia during the course of the disease. The second and third divisions of the fifth cranial nerve are the next involved, in which case the patient usually complains of numbness or pain on one side of the face. The frequency of neurological symptoms in patients with nasopharyngeal carcinoma is relatively high. In Chiang and Griem's (1973) series of 350 patients about 40 per cent complained of headache, 20 per cent of tinnitus, 20

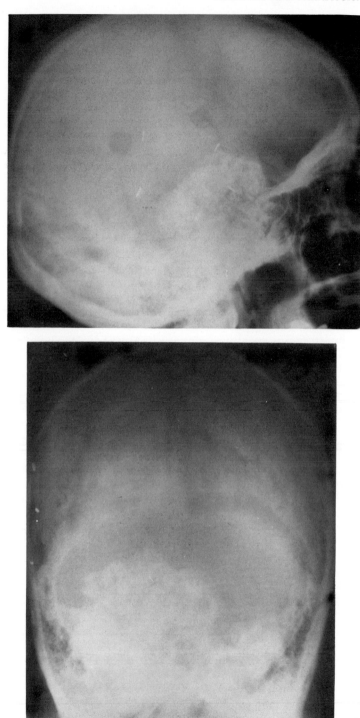

Figure 5.53. Massive mid-line calcification in a chordoma.

per cent of double vision and 12 per cent facial numbness. Thus with this type of clinical manifestation, which may be similar to that caused by a large pituitary tumour, special attention should be given to the radiological examination of the nasopharynx. Basal views of the skull and tomograms of the area suspected are mandatory. These may show bone destruction and soft tissue swelling which may be difficult to detect in other projections. The possibility of carcinoma arising primarily in the sphenoidal air sinus should also be considered. This is a rare lesion which may be difficult to differentiate from an invasive chromophobe adenoma (Figure 5.60).

Nasopharyngeal carcinoma extending postero-laterally from the pharyngeal recess and involving the lower cranial nerves, the ninth, tenth, eleventh and twelfth, is easier to diagnose because these patients usually complain of difficulty in swallowing and in phonation.

Mucocele of the sphenoid sinus

Sphenoid sinus mucoceles and pyoceles arise as a result of occlusion of the sinus ostium by chronic sinusitis, although cysts arising from goblet-cell glands may also be a cause. It is a potentially serious condition because it has been misdiagnosed and operated on as a pituitary tumour thereby increasing the morbidity and mortality of an otherwise curable disease. The frequency of misdiagnosing the lesion as a pituitary tumour has been emphasised by many authors (Bloom, 1965; Minagi, Margolis and Newton, 1972). As the sinus expands, the pressure is primarily transmitted to the thin bones forming the apices of the orbits and secondarily to the cavernous sinus and the floor of the sella. Thus headache, visual failure and ophthalmoplegia are common and pituitary insufficiency may occur. The sinus has been described expanding postero-laterally and presenting as a cerebello-pontine angle tumour (Phelps and Toland, 1969).

The main radiological findings are: (1) a well-defined soft tissue swelling within the sinus: (2) evidence of sphenoid sinus expansion and atrophy of its wall; (3) destruction of bony septa within the sinus; (4) bone destruction may extend into the optic foramen, the superior orbital fissure or the floor of the sella, depending on the vector of growth. In a review study of a large number of cases, involvement of the sella was present in more than 60 per cent (Nugent, Sprinkle and Bloor, 1970).

The sella in rhinitis 'caseosa'

This is a very rare chronic infective granulomatous condition which is more familiar to the ear, nose and throat surgeon than to the radiologist or neurosurgeon. It is characterised by the formation of masses of caseous material in the nose and often in the maxillary antra also. It may involve the sphenoidal air sinus and may cause destruction of the sella (Craig, 1961).

Sella enlargement in adult cretinism

Inadequately treated cases of cretinism may show enlargement of the pituitary fossa, perhaps the result of compensatory hypertrophy of the hypophysis. In a series of 32 adult cretins in whom therapy had been omitted or was inadequate at the critical stage of developing the disease, Middlemass (1959) found enlargement of the sella in about one-fifth of the cases.

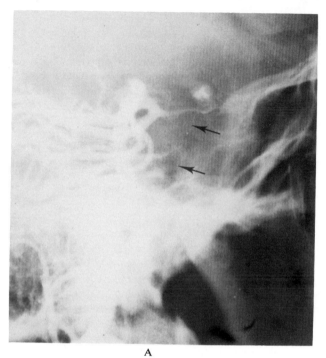

A

Figure 5.54A. Posterior displacement of the basilar artery by chordoma. Arrows point to ghost shadow of the clivus. Note abnormal curve of the basilar artery with a front concavity.

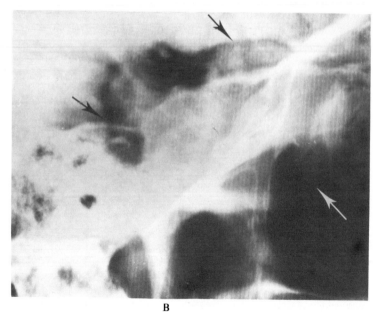

B

Figure 5.54B. Intracranial extension of chordoma outlined by air in the basal cisterns. Pneumoencephalogram, lateral view in brow-up position. The black arrows point to the upward extension of the tumour, white arrow to forward invasion into the nasopharynx.

CAVERNOUS SINUS VENOGRAPHY

Because of the close anatomical relation of the cavernous sinus to the pituitary fossa contrast visualisation of the sinuses may be valuable in the search for a pituitary neoplasm. Cavernous sinus venography will indicate the true extent of an intrasellar tumour that has not extended into the cerebral sub-arachnoid space. It has been shown that using this technique lateral extension of a pituitary tumour which was not shown at pneumoencephalography could be demonstrated (Hasso et al, 1975).

The technique of cavernous sinus venography is fully described elsewhere (Takahashi and Tanaka 1971). The sinuses can be visualised by injecting contrast medium directly into the supra-orbital or supratrochlear vein, or by catheterisation of the inferior petrosal sinus via the femoral vein, the brachial vein or the internal jugular vein. Each method of approach has its advantages, so that while one may fail to outline the sinus, the other may succeed. Small lesions indent the medial wall of the sinus and larger tumours may displace it laterally or obliterate its cavity.

BRAIN SCINTIGRAPHY

The radioactive isotope generally used for brain scanning is technetium 99m as pertechnetate. It has the advantages of being a pure gamma emitter (140 keV) with a relatively short half-life (6 hours). For an adult patient an intravenous dose of 10 to 15 mCi is given 2 to 4 hours before 'scanning'. To reduce the uptake of isotope by the choroid plexus, many workers prefer to give an oral dose of 200 to 1000 mg of potassium perchlorate before the examination. ^{99m} Tc is mainly excreted through the gastrointestinal tract and partly through the kidneys.

A solid sizeable tumour, which is not less than perhaps 2 cm in diameter, shows as a localised area of increased concentration of the radio-active isotope (Figure 5.61). In contrast, practically all avascular cystic lesions do not show on the brain scan − a point which is sometimes very helpful in differentiating between such lesions as cystic craniopharyngioma and pituitary adenoma. Similarly, an intrasellar tumour or a small suprasellar extension cannot be detected by brain scintigraphy. This is because they are masked by pools of circulating isotope in the vascular structures around the sella, the mucous membrane of the sphenoid sinus, the skull base and the superficial muscles. The value of isotope scanning in cases of pituitary and parapituitary tumours is therefore limited and should not be relied upon as a primary method of investigation.

COMPUTERISED TOMOGRAPHY

Computerised tomography (Ct or EMI scan) is a new x-ray technique in which the head is examined in a series of transverse slices of 8 or 13 mm thickness. Each slice is scanned from multiple directions in minute tissue blocks of $1.5 \times 1.5 \times 13$ or 8 mm. Through a system of x-ray detectors, photo-multipliers and a computer, the photons (x-ray units) absorbed by each block are calculated. The results which can be obtained on a print-out, are displayed on a cathode-ray tube and the image is photographed with a polaroid camera (Hounsfield, 1973). Tissues containing elements of high atomic number absorb more radiation and appear white, cerebrospinal fluid appears dark grey and other brain constituents, depending on their density, present different shades of grey (Figure 5.62).

This new technique has many merits and has been acclaimed as the most important invention since Roentgen's discovery of x-rays. It is much more sensitive than conventional

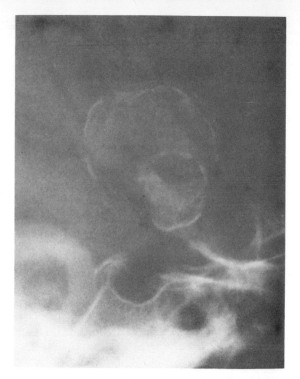

A

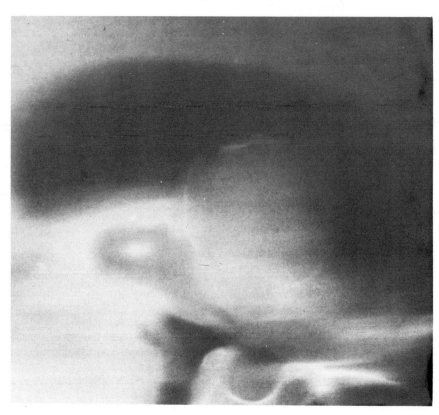

B

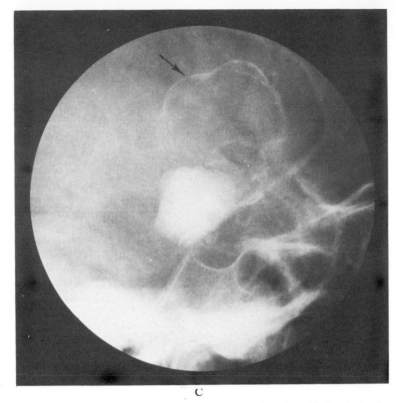

C

Figure 5.55. Massive berry aneurysm. A 62-year-old male patient was investigated for headache, dementia and bilateral papilloedema. Routine skull radiographs showed a large calcified ring above the sella (A). Air studies (ventriculography and pneumoencephalography) showed a large tumour abutting on the anterior wall of the third ventricle and bulging into the floor of both frontal horns (B). At angiography (C) this was shown to be an aneurysm most occupied by thrombus with mural calcification (arrow). Only a small portion of the aneurysm was filled with contrast medium.

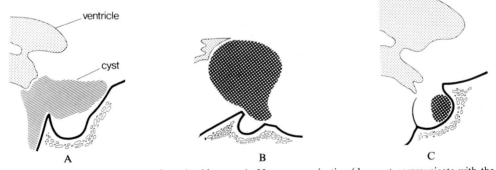

A   B   C

Figure 5.56. Three main types of arachnoid cysts. A. Non-communicating (does not communicate with the subarachnoid space) cyst. This type of cyst does not fill with air at pneumoencephalography. Thus, it is indistinguishable from other suprasellar tumours. Visual manifestations are minimal or absent but hypothalamic dysfunction may occur. B. Communicating suprasellar cyst. This type of cyst fills with air at pneumoencephalography. It leads to intermittent obstruction of the foramen of Monro, which is precipitated by forward bending, coughing or straining. C. Intrasellar arachnoid cyst. This is a rare cause of an enlarged pituitary fossa but does not appear to be clinically significant. This diagram is reproduced by kind permission of the editor of *Clinical Radiology*.

radiography. It does not require arterial puncture or the use of radio-active isotopes and the radiation dose (2 to 4 rads) is not greater than that received from routine skull radiographs. Computerised tomography readily outlines the ventricular system and it is the most decisive investigation in the diagnosis of brain haemorrhage and infarction. With few exceptions, practically any cerebral tumour is usually apparent on the Ct scan (Paxton and Ambrose, 1974). Unfortunately, this is not so in cases of pituitary and parapituitary tumours. Small lesions in the sellar region are usually masked by the overlying bone and are not revealed on the Ct scan. Large suprasellar lesions, on the other hand, are usually detectable and in them a histological diagnosis may be achieved.

The normal anatomy of the suprasellar cistern is shown in Figure 5.63. It is pentagonal in shape and within it the optic chiasm can be identified. Although failure to outline the cistern may be interpreted with suspicion in a patient who is being investigated for a pituitary lesion, the cistern, for technical reasons, may not be obvious on a normal scan. Pituitary adenoma appears as a well defined circular area which is slightly higher in density than the surrounding brain. Like many other lesions, its density may be enhanced following the intravenous injection of a large dose of a water soluble contrast medium (Figure 5.64). The appearance of craniopharyngioma on the Ct scan is different but often pathognomonic. It depends on the consistency of the lesion and its cholesterol and calcium content. Cholesterol, being less dense than water, appears very dark in colour in contrast to the whitish appearance of the tumour capsule. The latter is often contrast enhanced (Figure 5.65). Calcium flecks within the tumour may be apparent on the Ct scan even if they are not sufficiently dense to cast a shadow on the skull radiographs (Figure 5.66). The solid noncalcified craniopharyngioma has a density similar to the surrounding brain and cannot be differentiated from a malignant neoplasm. The author has seen only one such case and its density was not contrast enhanced (Figure 5.67).

Suprasellar meningioma, like pituitary adenoma, is a well-defined lesion but it is characterised by a remarkable increase in density following contrast enhancement (Figure 5.68). In fact, the tumour may appear so dense that it may be mistaken for a large berry aneurysm on the Ct scan alone (Figure 5.69). Another type of lesion which has been seen in the suprasellar region is optic chiasm glioma (Figure 5.70). In this case the tumour was very extensive; it was markedly contrast enhanced and its extension appeared to follow the radiation of the optic tract.

Although the illustrations provided here may appear fairly convincing, the author wishes to draw attention to the high incidence of false-negative results in cases of pituitary and parapituitary tumours, to the similarity between aneurysms and some tumours and to the possibility of coincidental aneurysms in the presence of pituitary tumours. At the present stage of its development, the Ct scan is a useful adjunctive investigation that shows the ventricular volume before an air study is contemplated. When positive, the Ct scan may reveal the pathology of the lesion and from the way the computer information is reconstructed, it provides an excellent illustration of the lateral extension of any intracranial neoplasm.

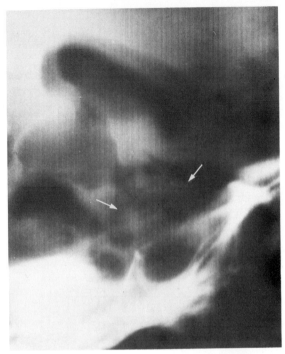

Figure 5.57. Non-communicating arachnoid cyst. A 17-year-old female patient was investigated for headache amenorrhoea and retarded skeletal maturity. Her visual acuity and fields were normal. The skull radiographs showed changes in the sella suggestive of a suprasellar tumour and angiography showed deformation of the anterior part of the circle of Willis in keeping with a suprasellar tumour which was confirmed on pneumoencephalography (arrows). This, at operation, was shown to be an arachnoid cyst.

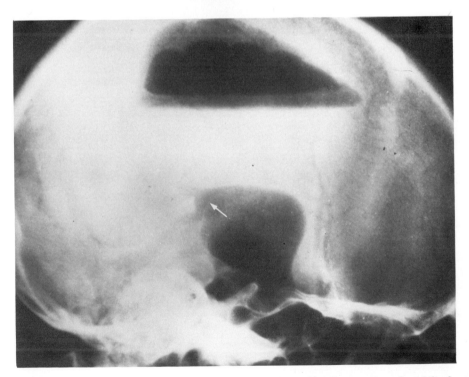

Figure 5.58. Communicating suprasellar arachnoid cyst. A 45-year-old patient was investigated for frontal headache which was precipitated by change of posture. At pneumoencephalography marked distention of the lateral ventricles was found. There was obstruction of the foramen of Monro due to a large suprasellar cyst which is delineated by a thin hair line membrane from the floor of the third ventricle (arrow). This case is reproduced by kind permission of Dr Sansregret and the editor of the *American Journal of Roentgenology*.

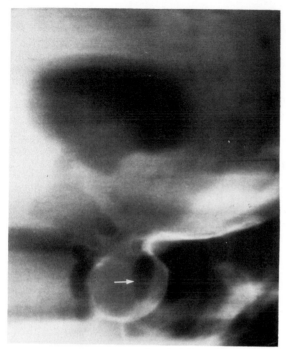

Figure 5.59. Intrasellar arachnoid cyst. A 46-year-old female patient was investigated for temporal lobe epilepsy. Skull radiographs showed an enlarged pituitary fossa. At pneumoencephalography this was shown to be due to arachnoid cyst within the sella (arrow) and had no relation to her symptoms. (By kind permission of the editor of *Clinical Radiology*)

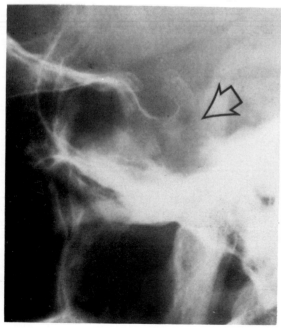

Figure 5.60. Carcinoma of the sphenoid sinus. Note: 1. bone destruction of the clivus, similar to chordoma (arrow). 2. erosion of the floor of the sella. 3. soft tissue swelling within the sinus.

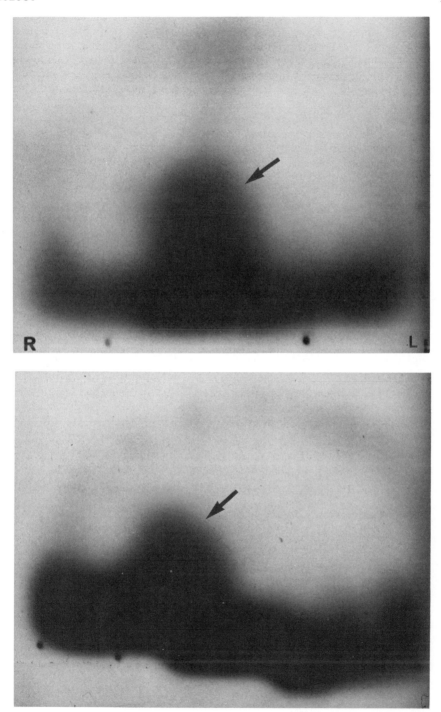

Figure 5.61. Brain scintigram (Tc 99m). Antero-posterior and lateral views of a massive pituitary adenoma (arrows).

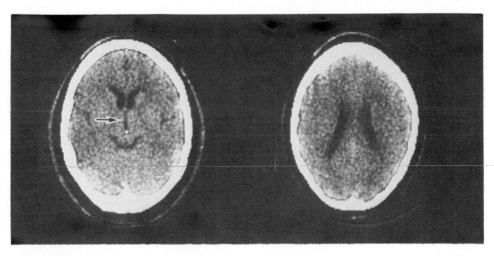

Figure 5.62. Normal Ct scan. Arrow points to the third ventricle.

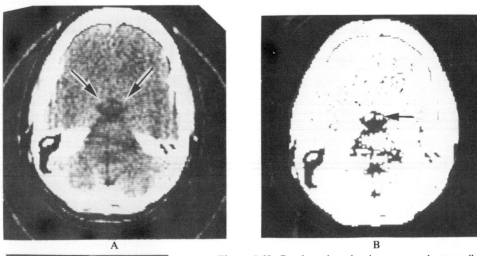

A   B

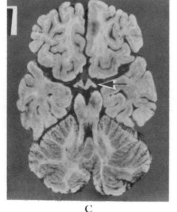

C

Figure 5.63. Basal section showing a normal suprasellar cistern (arrows in A). By altering the density control mechanisms on the machine, one is able to highlight the optic chiasm within the cistern (horizontal arrow in B). (C) is a brain section at approximately the same level for comparison.

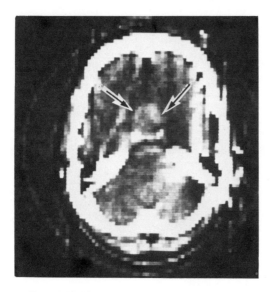

Figure 5.64. Pituitary adenoma (contrast enhanced).

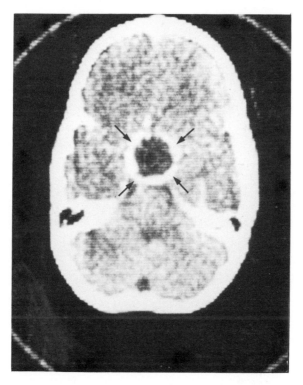

Figure 5.65. Cystic craniopharyngioma. The tumour capsule is contrast enhanced (arrows). Note the low density of cholesterol within the tumour. (By courtesy of Dr D. C. Harwood-Nash.)

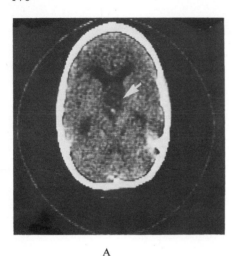

A

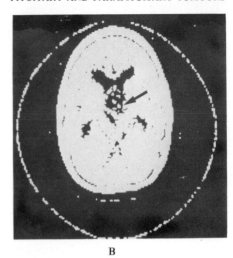

B

Figure 5.66. Calcium flecks. Arrow in (A) points to a cystic craniopharyngioma (contrast enhanced). The calcified spots are more apparent on (B) taken at different density control settings.

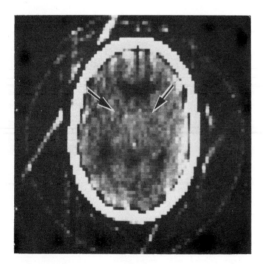

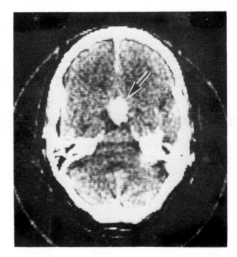

Figure 5.67. Solid craniopharyngioma (contrast enhanced). The tumour density (arrows) is similar to the surrounding brain and its margins cannot be outlined.

Figure 5.68. Suprasellar meningioma (contrast enhanced).

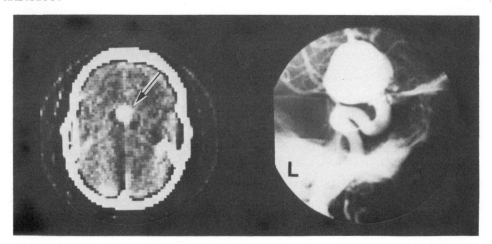

Figure 5.69. Berry aneurysm (contrast enhanced). Note the similarity of the lesion to suprasellar meningioma.

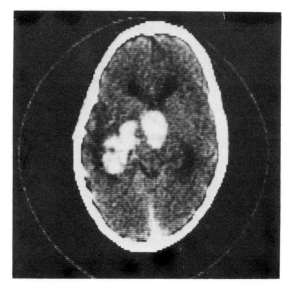

Figure 5.70. Optic chiasm glioma (contrast enhanced).

REFERENCES

Addy, D. P. & Hudson, F. P. (1972) Diencephalic syndrome of infantile emaciation: analysis of the literature and report of further three cases. *Archives of Disease in Childhood*, **47**, 338–343.

Ambrose, J. (1973) Radiological diagnosis of pituitary tumours. In *Pituitary Tumours*, pp. 79–121. London: Butterworths.

Banna, M. (1973) *Comprehensive Study of Craniopharyngioma*. MD thesis, Newcastle upon Tyne.

Banna, M. (1974) Arachnoid cysts in the hypophyseal area. *Clinical Radiology*, **25**, 323–326.

Banna, M., Schatz, S. W., Molot, M. J. and Groves, J. (1976) Primary intrasellar germinoma.

Bird, A. C., Nolan, B., Gargano, F. P. & David, N. J. (1970) Unruptured aneurysm of the supraclinoid carotid artery. *Neurology*, **20**, 445–454.

Block, M. A., Goree, J. A. & Jimenez, J. P. (1973) Craniopharyngioma with optic canal enlargement simulating glioma of the optic chiasm. *Journal of Neurosurgery*, **39**, 523–527.

Bloom, D. L. (1965) Mucoceles of the maxillary and sphenoid sinuses. *Radiology*, **85**, 1103–1110.

Brisman, R., Hughes, J. E. O. & Mount, L. A. (1969) Cerebrospinal fluid rhinorrhea and the empty sella. *Journal of Neurosurgery*, **31**, 538–543.

Bull, J. (1953) The radiological diagnosis of intracranial tumours in children. *Journal of the Faculty of Radiologists*, **4**, 149–170.

Bull, J. (1969) Massive aneurysms at the base of the brain. *Brain*, **92**, 535–570.

Bull, J. W. D. & Schunk, H. (1962) The significance of displacement of the cavernous portion of the internal carotid artery. *British Journal of Radiology*, **35**, 801–814.

Burrows, E. H. (1963) Bone changes in orbital neurofibromatosis. *British Journal of Radiology*, **36**, 549–561.

Burrows, E. H. (1964) The so-called J-sella. *British Journal of Radiology*, **37**, 661–669.

Chester, W. & Chester, E. M. (1940) The vertebral column in acromegaly. *American Journal of Roentgenology*, **44**, 552–557.

Chiang, T. C. & Griem, M. L. (1973) Nasopharyngeal cancer. *The Surgical Clinics of North America*, **53**:1, 121–133.

Coenegracht, J. M., De Bie, J. P. A. M., Coene, L. N. M. & Padberg, G. (1975) Deficiency of gonadotropin-releasing factor in a patient with hydrocephalus internus. *Journal of Neurosurgery*, **43**, 239–243.

Craig, O. (1961) Enlargement of the sphenoidal fissure and the sella by 'rhinitis caseosa'. *British Journal of Radiology*, **34**, 784–787.

Cushing, H. (1932) The basophil adenomas of the pituitary body and their clinical manifestations (Pituitary Basophilism). *Bulletin of Johns Hopkins Hospital*, **50**, 134–195.

Dahlin, D. C. & MacCarty, C. S. (1952) Chordoma. A study of 59 cases. *Cancer*, **5**, 1170–1178.

di Chiro, G. & Lindgren, E. (1952) Bone changes in cases of suprasellar meningioma. *Acta Radiologica*, **38**, 133–138.

di Chiro, G. & Nelson, K. B. (1962) The volume of the sella turcica. *American Journal of Roentgenology*, **87**, 989–1008.

Dodge, H. W. Jr, Love, J. G., Craig, W. Mck., Dockerty, M. B., Kearns, T. P., Holman, C. B. & Hayles, A. B. (1958) Gliomas of the optic nerves. *Archives of Neurology and Psychiatry*, **79**, 607–621.

du Boulay, G. (1957) The radiological evidence of raised intracranial pressure in children. *British Journal of Radiology*, **30**, 375–377.

du Boulay, G. H. & El-Gammal, T. (1966) The classification, clinical value and mechanism of sella turcica changes in raised intracranial pressure. *British Journal of Radiology*, **39**, 422–442.

du Boulay, G. H. & Trickey, S. E. (1962) Calcification in chromophobe adenoma. *British Journal of Radiology*, **35**, 793–795.

El-Gammal, T. & Allen, M. B. Jr. (1972) The intrasellar subarachnoid recess. *Acta Radiologica*, **13**, 401–412.

Evans, R. A., Schwartz, & Chutorian, A. M. (1963) Radiologic diagnosis in paediatric ophthalmology. *Radiologic Clinics of North America*, **1**, 459–495.

Farberov, B. J. (1937) Roentgenological diagnosis of the foramen opticum. *Acta Radiologica*, **18**, 594–606.

Fry, I. Kelsey & du Boulay, G. (1965) Some observations on the sella in old age and arterial hypertension. *British Journal of Radiology*, **38**, 16–22.

Gado, M. & Bull, J. W. D. (1971) The carotid angiogram in suprasellar masses. *Neuroradiology*, **2**, 136–153.

Girdwood, T. G. & Ross, E. M. (1969) The diencephalic syndrome of early infancy. *British Journal of Radiology*, **42**, 847–850.

Givner, I. (1945) Ophthalmologic features of intracranial chordoma and allied tumours of the clivus. *Archives of Ophthalmology*, **33**, 397–403.

Hasso, A. N., Bentson, J. R., Wilson, G. H. & Vignaud, J. (1975). Neuroradiology of the sphenoid region. *Radiology*, **114**, 619–627.

Holman, C. B. (1959) Roentgenologic manifestations of glioma of the optic nerve and chiasm. *American Journal of Roentgenology*, **82**, 462–471.

Hounsfield, G. N. (1973) Computarized transverse axial scanning (Tomography): Part 1. Description of System, **46**, 1016–1022.

Joplin, G. F. & Fraser, R. (1960) Quoted by Oon, C. L. (1960) *Ciba Foundation Colloquia on Endocrinology*, **13**, 14.

Kageyama, N. (1971) Ectopic pinealoma in the region of the optic chiasm. *Journal of Neurosurgery*, **31**, 670–675.

Kaufman, B. (1968) The 'empty' sella turcica – a manifestation of the intrasellar subarachnoid space. *Radiology*, **90**, 931–941.

Kaufman, B. & Chamberlin, W. B. Jr., (1972) The ubiquitous 'empty' sella turcica, *Acta Radiologica*, **13**, 413–425.

Kho, K. M., Wright, A. D., Doyle, F. H. (1970) Heel pad thickness in acromegaly. *British Journal of Radiology*, **43**, 119–125.

Kier, E. L. (1968) The infantile sella turcica: new roentgenologic and anatomic concepts based on a developmental study of the sphenoid bone. *American Journal of Roentgenology*, **102**, 747–767.

Knowlton, A. I. (1953) Cushing's syndrome. *Bulletin of the New York Academy of Medicine*, **29**, 441–465.

Krayenbühl, H. A. & Yasargil, M. G. (1968) *Cerebral angiography*. London: Butterworths.

Krieger, D. T., Krieger, H. P. & Soffer, L. J. (1964) Cushing's syndrome associated with suprasellar tumour. *Acta Endocrinologica*, **47**, 185–199.

Lee, W. M. & Adams, J. E. (1968) The empty sella syndrome. *Journal of Neurosurgery*, **28**, 351–356.

Lewtas, N. A. & Jefferson, A. A. (1966) The carotid cistern. A source of diagnostic difficulties with suprasellar extensions of pituitary adenomata. *Acta Radiologica*, **5**, 675–690.

Lowman, R. M., Robinson, F. & McAllister, W. B. (1964) The craniopharyngeal canal. *Acta Radiologica*, **5**, 41–53.

Mahmoud, M. E. (1958) The sella in health and disease. *British Journal of Radiology*, Suppl. 8.

Mascherpa, F. & Valantino, V. (1959) Intracranial calcification. pp. 25–27. Springfield, Illinois: Charles C. Thomas.

Mayer, E. G. (1959) Diagnose und differential diagnose in der Schädelröentgenologie. p. 375. Wien: Springer-Verlag.

Middlemass, I. B. D. (1959) Bone changes in adult cretins. *British Journal of Radiology*, **32**, 685–688.

Minagi, H. & Newton, T. H. (1969) Cartilaginous tumours of the skull base. *American Journal of Roentgenology*, **105**, 308–313.

Minagi, H., Margolis, T. & Newton, T. H. (1972) Tomography in the diagnosis of sphenoid sinus mucocele. *American Journal of Roentgenology*, **115**, 587–591.

Mortara, R. & Norrell, H. (1970) Consequences of a deficient sellar diaphragm. *Journal of Neurosurgery*, **32**, 565–573.

Murray, R. O. (1960) Radiological bone changes in Cushing's syndrome and steroid therapy. *British Journal of Radiology*, **33**, 1–19.

Nugent, G. R., Sprinkle, P. & Bloor, B. M. (1970) Sphenoid sinus mucoceles. *Journal of Neurosurgery*, **32**, 443–451.

Ommaya, A. K., di Chiro, G., Baldwin, M. & Pennybacker, J. B. (1968) Non-traumatic cerebrospinal fluid rhinorrhea. *Journal of Neurology, Neurosurgery and Psychiatry*, **31**, 214–225.

Oon, C. L. (1963) The size of pituitary fossa in adults. *British Journal of Radiology*, **42**, 845–847.

Paxton, R. & Ambrose, J. (1974) The EMI scanner. A brief review of the first 650 patients. *British Journal of Radiology*, **47**, 530–565.

Phelps, P. D. & Toland, J. A. (1969) Mucocoele of the sphenoidal sinus eroding the petrous temporal bone. *British Journal of Radiology*, **42**, 845-847.

Potter, G. D. & Trokel, S. L. (1971) Optic canal. In *Radiology of the Skull and Brain*, Vol. 1, pp. 487–540. St Louis: C. V. Mosby.

Powell, D. F., Baker, H. L. Jr & Laws, E. R. Jr (1974) The primary angiographic findings in pituitary adenomas. *Radiology*, **110**, 589–595.

Ross, R. J. & Greitz, T. V. B. (1966) Changes of the Sella turcica in chromophobic adenomas and eosinophilic adenomas. *Radiology*, **86**, 892–899.

Rovit, R. L. & Berry R. (1965) Cushing's syndrome and the hypophysis. *Journal of Neurosurgery*, **23**, 270–295.

Ruggiero, Giovanni (1966) Encephalography today. Refinements in technique and progress in diagnosis. *Acta Radiologica*, **5**, 705–715.

Sansregret, A., Le Doux, R., Duplantis, F., Lamoureux, C., Chapdelaine, A. & Leblanc, P. (1969) Suprasellar subarachnoid cysts. *American Journal of Roentgenology*, **105**, 291–297.

Schecter, M. M., Liebeskind, A. L. & Azar-Kia, B. (1974) Intracranial chordomas. *Neuroradiology*, **8**, 67–82.

Schuster, G. & Westberg, G. (1967) Gliomas of the optic nerve and chiasm. *Acta Radiologica*, **6**, 221–232.

Sherwood, M. (1953) The Troell-Junet syndrome. *Acta Radiologica*, **39**, 485–493.

Steinbach, H. L., Feldman, R. & Goldberg, M. B. (1959) Acromegaly. *Radiology*, **72**, 535–549.

Takahashi. M. & Tanaka, M. (1971) Cavernous sinus venography by transfemoral catheter technique. *Neuroradiology*, **3,** 1–3.

Taveras, J. M. & Wood, E. H. (1964) *Diagnostic Neuroradiology*. Baltimore: Williams and Wilkins.

Trapnell, D. H. & Bowerman, J. E. (1973) Dental manifestations of systemic disease, pp. 101–104. Butterworths & Co. Ltd.

Traub, S. P. (1961) *Roentgenology of Intracranial Meningiomas*, pp. 54–72. Springfield, Illinois: Charles C. Thomas.

Vezina, J. L. & Sutton, T. J. (1974) Prolactin-secreting pituitary microadenomas, roentgenologic diagnosis. *American Journal of Roentgenology*, **120,** 46–54.

Vidic, B. & Stom, D. (1968) The postnatal development of the sphenoidal sinus and its spread into the dorsum sellae and posterior clinoid processes. *American Journal of Roentgenology*, **104,** 177–193.

Weisberg, L. A., Housepian, E. M. & Saur, D. P. (1975) Empty sella syndrome as complication of benign intracranial hypertension. *Journal of Neurosurgery*, **43,** 177–180.

Wislocki, G. B. (1937) Meningeal relations of the hypophysis cerebri. *American Journal of Anatomy*, **61,** 95–130.

Wood, E. H. & Himadi, G. M. (1950) Chordomas: A roentgenologic study of 16 cases previously unreported. *Radiology*, **54,** 706–716.

CHAPTER SIX

Surgical Management

JOHN HANKINSON

As has been described in detail in Chapters 3 and 4 pituitary and parasellar tumours may produce visual disturbance by compression of the optic chiasm, nerves or tracts; endocrine hypofunction by compression of the hypophysis or hyperfunction by autonomous secretion; and occasionally, particularly in the craniopharyngiomas, hydrocephalus by obstruction of the foramina of Monro. Surgery, irradiation and hormonal replacement are the three therapeutic measures available. There can be little argument about replacement therapy and this is dealt with in Chapter 3. It would also be generally accepted that the introduction in 1950 of adrenal corticosteroids was the most significant advance in the surgical management of these tumours. The relationship between surgery and radiotherapy is more open to debate. There are three main problems: (1) the selection of those cases, if any, of pituitary adenoma, where radiotherapy alone is the treatment of choice; (2) the value of post-operative radiotherapy; and (3) the place of radiotherapy in the treatment of craniopharyngioma.

In about 1926, Harvey Cushing began to use post-operative irradiation therapy following operations for pituitary adenoma. The dosage was small and the technique in its early stages relatively inaccurate but, despite these factors, it was soon apparent that the recurrence rate in cases so treated was significantly smaller (at five years no recurrence had taken place in 65.3 per cent as against 32.8 per cent with the trans-sphenoidal operation and 87.1 per cent as against 57.5 per cent following craniotomy). Henderson (1939) in his analysis of Cushing's 338 pituitary tumour cases was convinced of the improvement in prognosis by post-operative irradiation. A tumour recurrence of approximately 13 per cent in the transfrontal operation followed by radiotherapy compares favourably to results achieved in more recent series with recurrence rates of about 7 per cent by similar techniques but with more sophisticated radiotherapy as reported by Ray and Patterson (1962) and Elkington and McKissock (1967). It is now the practice of the majority of neurosurgeons to refer their patients to the radiotherapist following surgery if radiation has not been given before surgery. But what of the more difficult question of the use of radiotherapy as the treatment of choice, surgery being invoked in a minority of cases where radiotherapy is judged to have failed?

Radiotherapy as an alternative to surgery in the treatment of pituitary tumours has been favoured predominantly, but not by any means universally, by surgeons in the United States and paradoxically has been most successfully developed and persuasively described by the neurosurgeons of the Lahey Clinic, a group long famous for surgical prowess.

Horrax (1958) regards the introduction of megavoltage therapy in 1950 as the crucial factor in the effective and safe handling of these lesions by irradiation as the primary treatment. He found that initially about 60 per cent of patients receiving previous radiation had to be operated on because radiation alone was not effective. At the time of his report of the patients receiving megavoltage therapy only 12 per cent had to undergo surgery to retain adequate vision. In 1962 Davidoff, explaining his attitude to this problem, stated that 'unless the patient has an immediate threat to his vision, unless the diagnosis of pituitary adenoma is not absolutely certain, unless the radiation therapy is not effective — i.e., the radiation therapy is followed by further deterioration of vision — we treat with radiation first, and if radiation fails, then we use surgery. In other cases we use surgery at the start.' There can be no argument against radiotherapy and its alleged but admittedly rare complications as most neurosurgeons will make use of it after surgery.

The object of irradiation as an alternative to surgery is, of course, to avoid the risks of intracranial operation. Ray and Patterson (1962) report no operative mortality in 85 pituitary operations performed on 80 patients between the years 1950 and 1960. Two hundred and sixty cases described by Elkington and McKissock showed an overall mortality rate at operation and within the subsequent six weeks of 10 per cent. Among the 45 patients (18 per cent of the total) with large or extensive tumours the operative mortality rate was 33 per cent, while among the remainder it was just under 5 per cent. Similar figures are quoted by G. Jefferson (1940) and Bakay (1950). A. A. Jefferson (1969) reported a personal series in which there was a 33 per cent mortality in 'massive' suprasellar extensions. The advantages of the surgical procedure are the greater certainty of diagnosis and hence indications for treatment and the more expeditious relief of chiasmal compression. In practice both groups observe a reasonable spirit of compromise, as exemplified by the exceptions to the rule given above by Davidoff. Similarly it may well be prudent to withhold surgery and to give a trial of irradiation in the poor surgical risk case and in those showing radiological evidence of a massive suprasellar extension of the tumour. It should perhaps be mentioned that the modern trans-sphenoidal operation may well alter the attitude of surgeons to the two groups of cases just described, which will be considered later in this chapter.

The treatment of craniopharyngiomas has proved a disappointing experience for most neurosurgeons. Radical surgery has been the policy of only one group (Matson and Crigler, 1960, 1969) and the attitude towards palliative surgery and radiotherapy varies from scepticism (Ingraham and Matson, 1954) to enthusiasm (Kramer, Southard and Mansfield, 1968). Again it seems that the technical improvements in both surgery and radiotherapy render much that has been written on this subject in the past irrelevant to the present situation. With the use of modern anaesthetic techniques, cortisone and magnification, more of these tumours can be removed completely with acceptable mortality and morbidity rates and equally, following incomplete surgery, megavoltage therapy can deliver adequate irradiation sufficiently accurately for safety.

PRE-OPERATIVE ASSESSMENT AND MANAGEMENT

In these cases pituitary inadequacy is usually partial only. Lack of gonadotrophins is usually evident but is often isolated and inadequate adrenal function is rare in patients coming to surgery. Indeed children with little pituitary function may have adequate independent adrenal and thyroid activity. When inadequate adrenal function is suspected from lassitude, low blood pressure and low serum sodium it will have previously been confirmed by measurements of cortisol levels and by other tests described in Chapter 3. In such cases if operation is not urgently indicated replacement therapy should be undertaken for at least two weeks before major surgery. However, other investigations such as carotid angiography and air encephalography can be safely carried out during this period of replacement therapy. If there is no evidence of adrenal insufficiency no replacement is required before surgery and cortisone or hydrocortisone should not be given until the day of operation. Thyroid deficiency, when present, is often minimal and may easily be overlooked, particularly the protein-bound iodine (PBI) and radio-iodine uptake may be within normal limits. Eyebrow loss, excess weight, lassitude and low basal body temperature are indicative of serious thyroid deficiency. Again if deficiency is thought to exist and operation is not urgent two weeks' replacement therapy should precede definitive operation. If operation is urgent L-thyroxine should be given as soon as the deficiency is recognised, provided that cortisol deficiency, if present, has also been corrected (see Chapter 3). The occurrence of diabetes insipidus due to ADH lack in the presence of ACTH is extremely rare with a pituitary adenoma, although it is found as a presenting symptom in one-quarter of the cases of craniopharyngioma in childhood.

ANAESTHESIA AND OPERATIVE MANAGEMENT

No special anaesthetic techniques are indicated. For intracranial procedures premedication and anaesthesia are as for other craniotomies. In this clinic all patients are placed in the head-up position and are slightly over-ventilated ($PaCO_2$ 25 to 30 mm Hg) during surgery. In cases not receiving pre-operative replacement hydrocortisone 100 mg is given by intramuscular injection with the premedication or as soon as the patient is anaesthetised.

Occasionally a considerable diuresis starts during the operation and patients should be catheterised shortly after induction and urine output measured. It has never been found necessary to give pitressin during the operation in the author's series of cases. Since these patients will require intravenous infusions for at least three days post-operatively more than usual care should be taken to establish an intravenous line. Skin over the vein puncture is swabbed with iodine and a strictly aseptic cannulation is performed. In children or those with poor peripheral veins an inferior vena cava cannula is introduced through the saphenous vein by cut-down in the groin. This allows the taking of blood samples as well as infusions.

POST-OPERATIVE MANAGEMENT

Corticosteroid cover is given routinely. Our regimen consists of 100 mg 6 hourly for 48 hours followed by 50 mg 6 hourly for 48 hours followed by 25 mg 6 hourly for 2 days followed by 25 mg b.d. This regimen probably provides more steroids than is necessary. We have seen no ill effects from it except in one woman who had mild hypomania which disappeared when the steroids were reduced.

Unsuspected thyroid deficiency may be revealed in the post-operative period. This is shown by prolonged drowsiness or stupor and sometimes by a subnormal body temperature in the presence of a normal or raised blood pressure and adequate corticosteroid cover. This is treated with 60 to 80 μg of triiodothyronine i.v. daily for 48 hours with the simultaneous administration of 0.1 mg L-thyroxine daily by mouth or stomach tube. The response to this can be dramatic but the risk of coronary thrombosis during treatment of myxoedema must be borne in mind. Long-term thyroid replacement should be assessed two to three weeks post-operatively.

ADH deficiency may not be manifest until 12 to 48 hours post-operatively. It is related to retraction in the region of the supra-optic nucleus rather than to ablation of the posterior pituitary. It is common after operations for craniopharyngioma and rare after operations for chromophobe or eosinophilic tumours. In patients showing an abnormal diuresis the following regimen is followed. Electrolytes are measured at least 12 hourly. Urine output is measured hourly and in adults aqueous pitressin, 5 units, is given subcutaneously whenever the hourly output excedes 150 ml. (For children the dose and output are scaled down appropriately.) Intravenous replacement is adjusted to maintain fluid balance with 500 ml of dextrose in one-quarter N-saline to 1000 ml of N-saline, 0.5 g of potassium being added to each 500 ml unit. This regimen is then modified as the serum electrolyte pattern suggests.

Oestrogen or testosterone replacement may be indicated in adults. There is no indication for these hormones in children, least of all in those unlikely ever to reach adulthood or adult social adjustment. Some patients may require long-term anabolic steroid treatment to counteract loss of lean body mass. Eosinophilic tumours are associated with a raised blood sugar and insulin resistance. We have never found this a clinically significant problem.

Occasionally patients with large lateral extensions of chromophobe tumours have epileptiform attacks pre-operatively. These patients are treated as others with focal epilepsy. Rarely a patient is seen in whom the first convulsion is in the immediate post-operative period.

SURGICAL PROCEDURES

Surgical procedures fall into the following four groups. The indications for each procedure will be considered and although any given case would be more appropriately treated by one procedure than another, it is unlikely that they all appear in the repertoire of most neurosurgeons or indeed in the repertoire of any neurosurgeon.
1. Intracranial — transfrontal approach.
2. Intracranial — temporal approach.
3. Trans-sphenoidal surgical.
4. Trans-sphenoidal — interstitial irradiation.

Transfrontal craniotomy was used by Cushing in his early cases but subsequently a greater proportion of cases were treated by the trans-sphenoidal operation. The modern transfrontal craniotomy differs only in certain details from the original operation but improvements in anaesthetic and other techniques have greatly eased operative exposure and added greatly to the patient's safety. The skin incision may be a unilateral frontal incision of classical shape in which the anterior part of the medial limb can be seen in front of the hair-line. Or the scalp incision can be hidden within the hair-line either by employing Dandy's concealed hypophyseal incision or by a coronal skin incision which is entirely within the hair-line. In any case it is essential that the frontal bone should be exposed as low as the floor of the anterior fossa just above the superciliary ridge, if necessary by opening the frontal sinus. A sufficiently low exposure greatly assists visualisation of the tumour area and reduces retraction of the frontal lobe. Cosmetic considerations also suggest that any burr holes made under the visible part of the frontal scalp should be filled in at the end of the operation, either by some special plastic button, or more readily with bone dust. This avoids the very obvious depression of the scalp which otherwise results. As long as the anterior bony cut is made sufficiently low the quadrilateral bone flap itself needs to be of only moderate dimensions. With modern anaesthesia it is unlikely that a pituitary tumour would be associated with raised intracranial pressure and so it is not often that the necessity for aspirating the anterior horn of the lateral ventricle arises. It is commoner now to elevate the frontal lobe after incising the dura anteriorly and as far laterally as just beyond the pterion but this used to be done by an extradural approach over the orbital plate and the dura was incised along the lesser wing of the sphenoid. This protected the undersurface of the frontal lobe from retraction but reduced the exposure. It must be confessed that the ease of retraction produced by modern anaesthesia in such cases increases the risk to the olfactory nerves as it is all too easy to damage the nerve on the operated side by traction and it is essential to protect the opposite olfactory nerve.

The question of the side upon which to approach a pituitary tumour gives rise to some discussion. A right-handed surgeon should employ a right-sided craniotomy and the opposite is the case for a left-handed surgeon. This is only superseded if the clinical presentation, particularly the visual field charts and the radiological studies have indicated that the tumour is situated predominantly on one side. The temporal approach to pituitary tumours was used by Horsley (1906) in ten cases and it was suggested by Jefferson (1957) that his preference for the temporal route was a consequence of Horsley's experiences in experimental work on the pituitary in the dog and the monkey.

He evidently obtained a good view of the pituitary fossa from the side and described it using a small rhinoscopic mirror to inspect the interior of the sella, stating that he had an excellent view of the second and third nerves, of the crus cerebri and of the cavernous sinus. Eventually this approach to the pituitary region was almost completely abandoned in favour of the transfrontal approach. However, according to Poppen (1959) it is still the procedure of choice when there is clinical or radiological evidence of extension beyond the region of the sella and optic chiasm to the middle fossa, the third ventricle or to the interpeduncular fossa. In particular, it was recommended by Poppen as a possible solution of the difficult posteriorly extending pituitary tumour in the presence of a pre-fixed chiasm. Poppen feels that the decision as to which approach is indicated can be assisted by the radiological evidence. If the anterior cerebral arteries are displaced posteriorly and upwards with only slight opening of the carotid siphon, the anterior or frontal approach is indicated. If the posterior clinoid process is eroded and the anterior clinoids are reasonably normal, with little or no undercutting of the tuberculum sellae, and the angiograms show considerable opening of the carotid siphon, the temporal approach is more likely to give an adequate exposure of the tumour. With these criteria, therefore, the tumours most favourable to this approach include: craniopharyngiomas, adenomas, chordomas and meningiomas of the upper portion of the clivus and the dorsum sellae, as well as the large pituitary adenomas with a pre-fixed chiasm.

The lateral approach is through an opening in the anterior portion of the squamous temporal bone and, as with the transfrontal approach, it is essential to take the exposure as low as possible, in this case to the floor of the middle fossa. Occasionally it may be necessary to extend the posterior limb of a frontal incision down to the level of the zygoma and by removing temporal bone to achieve a lateral approach. The bone removed should include the lateral end of the sphenoidal ridge. Intracranial pressure is controlled by the usual manoeuvres of over-ventilation, dehydration or ventricular aspiration and the head is tilted in such a way as to allow the temporal lobe to lift from the floor of the middle fossa. Occasionally it is justified to sacrifice the antero-inferior portion of the temporal lobe. As with the transfrontal approach the interior of a pituitary adenoma is removed, usually by suction, but occasionally the use of rongeurs and a spoon is necessary. Extra nodules of tumour pressing on the optic pathways are removed and also pieces of capsule which seem to be causing any pressure, but no attempt is made to remove capsule which is adherent either to the optic nerves and chiasm or to the carotid artery or its branches. Post-operative irradiation will deal with any remaining pieces of tumour. A similar intra-capsular removal is used in the treatment of chordoma with subsequent removal of capsule as proves practicable. It is usually possible to perform a more radical removal of meningiomas in this situation except for those portions which sometimes surround the great vessels and cannot be safely removed and a similar situation sometimes occurs in relation to meningiomas around the optic nerve at the optic foramen. The third nerve is particularly sensitive to any interference and a partial or complete third nerve palsy will almost inevitably follow any manoeuvres which involve manipulation of the third nerve. Fortunately, this frequently recovers fairly rapidly in the post-operative period. Similarly the fourth nerve can be disturbed if the tentorial edge is incised and particularly if the diathermy is used on any bleeding points at the tentorial edge.

The Trans-sphenoidal Operation

The writings of Hirsch on this subject span the modern neurosurgical period (Hirsch, 1910, 1956, 1959). This was a technique much favoured by Cushing and indeed three-quarters of the 338 operations performed by him for pituitary adenomas were done by this route (Henderson, 1939). Although the intracranial operation increased in popularity in the intervening years, Hirsch and subsequently Hamlin (1962) in the United States, Dott and Guiot continued to use the method extensively and it was Guiot and Thibaut (1959) who introduced radiofluoroscopic control into the technique of the operation. Subsequently Hardy (1969, 1974) added the technique of microneurosurgery and has written extensively on the subject, particularly in relation to the surgery of hypersecreting pituitary tumours by the trans-sphenoidal route. Thus the basic technique and the arguments in its favour have remained practically unchanged since the early years of the century but great improvements have resulted in the use of the modern techniques of operative radiological screening and the development of the operating microscope and its associated armamentarium of fine instruments.

Guiot stresses the different therapeutic problems presented by the secreting and the non-secreting pituitary adenomas based essentially on their differing response to radiotherapy. Thus, while the pressure effects of the chromophobe adenoma can be satisfactorily controlled by a combination of surgical decompression and radiotherapy, the endocrine effects of the secreting adenomas, because of their relative resistance to irradiation, demand complete surgical extirpation. Guiot regards the following as indications for the trans-sphenoidal operation:
1. Old age or poor general medical condition.
2. Very severe bilateral impairment of vision.
   There seems no doubt that in such cases the chances of restitution of vision are greater by a trans-sphenoidal approach than by an intracranial approach because of the protection from even minimal surgical trauma by the diaphragma sellae when the approach is made from below.
3. With the invasive adenomas, particularly involving the sphenoid.
4. Retrochiasmal lesions in the presence of a pre-fixed chiasm when air encephalography has shown that there is no marked constriction between the intrasellar and suprasellar portions of the tumour.

Guiot considers the trans-sphenoidal operation contra-indicated when the presence of a narrow neck between the two portions of the adenoma has been demonstrated radiologically. This state of affairs occurred in about 10 per cent of his cases; in 28 per cent he regarded the indications as strongly suggesting the desirability of the trans-sphenoidal approach and in the remaining 62 per cent in his opinion either method would be suitable. The safety of this approach seems unquestionable, particularly with the use of antibiotic cover and the avoidance of secondary infection which occurred more frequently in the past. Because of this its advocates would, of course, use the trans-sphenoidal route much more frequently than in the cases regarded as being absolutely indicated.

Technique

Hardy regards the pituitary adenoma expanding inferiorly and causing enlargement of the floor of the sella turcica as the ideal indication for complete removal through this route, a view which has been held by many surgeons since Cushing described the operation in 1914. Similarly suprasellar extensions of moderate degree can be dealt with from below if the consistency of the tumour is diffluent or semi-liquid. For larger and more difficult suprasellar extensions the use of televised radiofluoroscopy to control the position of the instruments in the suprasellar area is an essential part of the modern trans-sphenoidal operation. An earlier and equally important technical development was the use of the operating microscope and its associated special instruments. Thus it has been possible to achieve selective removal of small intrapituitary adenomas with preservation of the normal pituitary tissue. Thus some cases of hyperpituitarism presenting with Cushing's syndrome, acromegaly, malignant exophthalmos or galactorrhoea have been treated successfully without the production of panhypopituitarism.

The operation as described by Hardy (1971) is performed under peroral endotracheal anaesthesia with the pharyngeal cavity packed with moist sponges to prevent aspiration. The patient is placed in the semi-sitting position with a portable image intensifier so positioned that the horizontal beam is centred on the sella turcica. The television screen is placed just behind and above the head of the patient so that the surgeon can look at the screen in line with the eye piece of the microscope (Figure 6.1). Radiofluoroscopic control is used as required during the operative procedure but only a few seconds of radiation

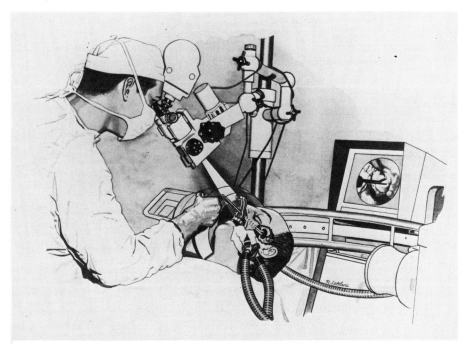

Figure 6.1. Trans-sphenoidal pituitary surgery using operating microscope and image intensifier with television screen. (By permission of Dr Hardy and the editor of the *Journal of Neurosurgery*).

exposure are necessary at each stage of the operation in order to ensure accurate placement of the instruments in the sella turcica.

A horizontal incision is made underneath the upper lip at the junction of the gum and the inner aspect of the lip extending to the canine fossa on either side. The incised upper lip is then elevated exposing the nasal bony cavity. After removal of the anterior nasal spinous process the mucosa of the floor of the nose is elevated as well as its reflection on both sides of the nasal septum. This is easily done as the mucosa has been partially detached by previous procaine infiltration. The inferior third of the anterior cartilaginous septum is then resected with a swivel knife exposing the vomer which has the appearance of the keel of a ship.

To obtain a wider operative field the sharp edge of the maxillary ridge and its lateral ascending branches should be sheared off and this will also assure a better grip for the serrated nasal speculum which is now inserted and opened to its maximal position. Thus the mucosal cavity is mobilised and the entire floor of the sphenoidal sinus is exposed. The vomer is then removed with grasping forceps or a sphenoid punch rongeur. The occasional thick, or 'acromegalic' vomer is excised piecemeal with a gouge. Further resection of the anterior aspect of the floor of the sinus gives a wide exposure of the whole cavity. The thin mucosa of the sinus is penetrated and deflected and any bony septa are removed until the posterior aspect of the sinus is widely exposed and the floor of the sella identified and its boundaries carefully located under direct vision and also with fluoroscopic control. The upper limit of the opening to be made is defined by the upper recess beneath the tuberculum sellae and laterally palpation with a blunt instrument defines a groove formed by the bulge of the carotid artery within the carotid canals on either side. At this stage the binocular microscope is placed in position for illumination of the operative cavity. The foregoing is an account of the trans-septal approach to the sphenoidal sinus and thence to the sella. Some surgeons prefer the trans-ethmoidal approach or a combination of trans-septal and trans-ethmoidal (Bateman, 1963). The advocates of the trans-ethmoidal approach maintain that this provides better exposure and a more direct access to the pituitary gland or the adenomas arising within it. Judging purely on results the uninvolved observer is not convinced of the superiority of one approach over the other.

Usually, with the downward displacement of the floor of the sella, when the sphenoid has been opened the sinus is seen to be partially or completely filled by the ballooned sella floor. The already thin floor is easily opened to produce a large window into the sella cavity. The dural lining of the sella will also be found to have been thinned by pressure of the tumour. The fluid contents of the adenoma are aspirated by needle puncture and thereafter the dura is incised in a cruciate fashion with the production as a rule of a large quantity of greyish, purple gelatinous tissue from the adenoma which fills the sphenoidal sinus and is removed by aspiration. Hardy stresses that other than the previously opened dura there is no capsule to a pituitary adenoma and no attempt should be made to remove what is thought to be a capsule as this is in continuity with the lateral wall of the sella and forms the inner aspect of the cavernous sinus and above the diaphragma sellae. Any more solid parts of the adenoma are removed with Ray's malleable curettes or Cushing's spoons. As a result of the normal intracranial pulsations the diaphragma sellae or the suprasellar extension spontaneously collapses into the sella. If this does not occur curettes are introduced under televised radiofluoroscopy and the suprasellar mass is detached piecemeal until the diaphragm is seen bulging downwards into the sella. The management of the suprasellar extension is greatly facilitated by the use of per-operative lumbar air encephalography. This is a natural consequence of the use of the image intensifier and is achieved by inserting a catheter into the lumbar subarachnoid space prior to operation.

In five per cent of Hardy's cases the adenoma was fibrous and removal was only possible by the use of the electrocautery loop. Cerebrospinal fluid leak is uncommon following trans-sphenoidal surgery since the distention of the tumour has produced adhesions of the diaphragm to the arachnoid with obliteration of the subarachnoid space. The diaphragm is thus a natural protection against fistula formation and it should not be penetrated when outlined by radiofluoroscopic control. Antibiotic powder is left in the sphenoidal cavity and the nasal mucosa is re-approximated with endonasal packs which are removed after 24 hours. Catgut sutures are used to re-approximate the gingival mucosa. There is thus no visible scar following this procedure. The scar by the medial side of the orbit for the trans-ethmoidal operation very rapidly becomes inconspicuous. The patient is given oral fluids six hours after the end of the anaesthetic and resumes normal diet the following morning. Ampicillin, 500 mg 6 hourly, is given for 24 hours prior to operation and is continued for five days thereafter.

Results of Surgery

Surgical results in this condition can be considered under three headings: mortality, visual improvement and recurrence of symptoms. The size of a pituitary tumour significantly influences the risks of surgical treatment. Thus Jefferson (1969) had a two per cent mortality for 'small adenomas in 98 patients and 33 per cent mortality in 12 patients with significant suprasellar extensions.' A large suprasellar extension was defined as one which when viewed on the lateral air encephalogram covered an area of more than 7.0 cm^2 or extended to within 6 mm of the foramen of Monro. Results of the early series of operations by Cushing, and subsequently of Cairns and Olivecrona gave mortality rates of the order of six and eight per cent for chromophobe adenomas but the rates were significantly higher in acromegaly. In 1962 Ray and Patterson reported a consecutive series of 85 operations by the transfrontal route without mortality. The clinical records of 221 cases of pituitary adenoma treated between 1955 and 1972 at Newcastle General Hospital were studied. A further 23 cases were excluded because they had been lost to follow-up or the clinical notes were considered inadequate. Their ages ranged from 17 to 77, there were slightly more females and the maximum incidence was in the fifth decade in both sexes. Chromophobe adenoma was diagnosed in 130, 85 suffered from acromegaly and 6 from Cushing's disease. There were 120 operations for pituitary adenoma of which only eight were in acromegalics (the majority of acromegalics during this period were given radiotherapy; see Chapter 7); eight deaths occurred (6.66 per cent) associated with the operation. Two deaths were due to myocardial infarction, three to 'brain swelling', two were attributed to haemorrhage at the time of operation and one with 'endocrine insufficiency' died two weeks after operation before the routine use of cortisone. It seems as if adrenal insufficiency predisposed the patient to cerebral oedema following operation. The use of cortisone at the time of operation has probably not greatly reduced the mortality rate but it has certainly improved the post-operative period, reduced the occasions on which the wound has been re-explored for cerebral oedema and has encouraged surgeons to be more radical in their removal of the adenoma.

Improvement of vision after operation

Of the 221 cases in the Newcastle series 125 showed some impairment of vision. Of these only 15 showed normal visual acuity in association with field defects. The symptoms in these cases were of less than six months duration and they all made a complete recovery of visual fields after treatment. Few patients had immediate improvement after operation, although subjective improvement of vision was often claimed within a few days of operation. Recovery of vision spread over several months and in a few cases improvement continued for 18 months but at the end of two years little further improvement can be expected. The speed of recovery was most rapid in the first six weeks and thereafter the rate of recovery diminished. In general it can be said that the less extensive and the more recent the visual impairment, the greater was the chance of successful treatment both in terms of acuity and in visual fields. As shown in Table 6.1, 63 of 117 patients, i.e., 53.8 per cent, showed complete recovery of function after operation and in all 101 of 117 patients, i.e. 86.3 per cent, showed some improvement of vision. Loss of visual acuity and visual field were never symmetrical but in ten cases after treatment visual acuity had returned to normal but a permanent field defect remained. Similarly in certain cases, visual function had returned to normal in one eye but showed only partial improvement or no improvement at all in the other eye, i.e., the more seriously affected eye. These cases have been considered to show only partial improvement. In the majority of patients the field defect was bitemporal but a few cases showed atypical and asymmetrical field loss and none of these cases obtained complete recovery of visual function.

Table 6.1. Visual function after treatment.

Duration of visual symptoms	No. of cases	Complete recovery	Partial recovery	Static	Worse	Not tested
0—6 months	53	38	11	1	1	2
7—12 months	30	18	7	1	2	2
13—18 months	8	3	2	2	1	0
19—24 months	14	2	8	3	0	1
More than 24 months	20	2	10	4	1	3
	125	63	38	11	5	8

Recovery from gross impairment of vision has been poor. Of 29 patients, 26 had gross impairment of vision in one eye and three in both eyes. Of ten patients capable of 'counting fingers' only, only one who had had symptoms for three months obtained complete recovery of vision but seven showed some significant improvement. Of four patients who could appreciate hand movements only, one returned to normal acuity but was left with a serious permanent field defect, two were unchanged and one improved to 6/36 at the end of six months. There were eight patients with perception of light only. Two regained some degree of useful vision, one improved to 'hand movements' only and five showed no improvement at all. Ten patients were blind either in one or both eyes and of these four suddenly became blind due to 'apoplexy'. Two regained useful vision and of the remaining six patients only one had any improvement in vision. Five patients remained totally blind in one eye. It appeared, therefore, that unless vision is at least 'finger counting' the prognosis as far as improvement in vision is concerned is very poor.

Recurrence

Fourteen patients were readmitted with symptoms of recurrence. At re-operation one showed the appearances of an empty sella, secondary to irradiation, with the optic nerves drawn into the fossa by adherence to the retracted diaphragm. Another patient, originally operated on in 1958, was re-explored in 1962 for failing vision but adhesions only were found. He was again operated on in 1969 and a cyst containing bloody fluid was partially removed. There was, however, no histological evidence of recurrence.

Of the remaining 12 patients tumour recurrence was demonstrated at operation in all but one, a 72-year-old man in whom symptoms had recurred 11 years after the first operation. He was given a course of irradiation, his symptoms regressed and he has remained well for six years. Only one of the recurrent cases had received irradiation after the original operation. This patient was readmitted within six months and at the second operation was found to have an invasive tumour and died one month later. The 11 cases of tumour recurrence, who had not had irradiation after operation, were members of a group of 18 treated in this way, all before 1960.

BROMOCRIPTINE TREATMENT

This recently developed derivative of ergot (2-brom-ergokryptine, CB154) suppresses prolactin secretion by direct action on the pituitary. Galactorrhoea associated with a pituitary adenoma ceases with doses of the drug of 7.5 to 15 mg daily. It may be that this would be the treatment of choice, avoiding pituitary injury by surgery or radiotherapy, if such a patient wished to become pregnant, but the probable rapid increase in size of an adenoma during pregnancy would have to be borne in mind. The suppression of prolactin secretion will often permit the ovaries to respond normally once more to LH and FSH.

Bromocriptine reduces growth hormone levels in most acromegalic patients, which is the opposite of its effect in normal people, and it is a most important development in the treatment of this condition. Reports of treatment to date are for periods of less than one year but in 20 per cent reduction in growth hormone levels has been sufficient to produce regression of clinical features. Dosage has been higher than those effective in hyperprolactinaemia and is usually between 20 and 60 mg daily. A combination of radiotherapy and bromocriptine may prove effective in cases resistant to either therapy alone. Advances can be expected, not only with combined therapy, but in the development of new ergot derivatives with even more specific effects. An account of bromocriptine and its bibliography is given in a leading article in the *British Medical Journal* of 20.12.1975, Volume **iv,** page 667.

PITUITARY APOPLEXY

Chromophobe and eosinophil adenomas sometimes give rise to a sudden, severe illness due to haemorrhage or infarction within their substance. The picture is similar to aneurysmal subarachnoid haemorrhage with sudden blindness or severe visual deterioration often associated with paralysis of ocular nerves. The diagnosis may become apparent when the appearances and history of endocrine disturbance combine with the appropriate radiological abnormalities. The practical danger is the acute onset of adrenal failure, which must be quickly recognised and effectively treated. Uihlein, Balfour and Donovan (1957) cite 71 cases from the literature of which 35 were acute and accounted for 21 deaths. In the past such devastating adrenal insufficiency denied patients the benefit of surgical decompression. Now with adequate intravenous replacement speedy de-compression is indicated, either by the frontal or sphenoidal route. A similar state of affairs, calling for the same plan of treatment, results from an acute ischaemic infarction of the adenoma. Zervas and Mendelson (1975) report three cases treated by stereotaxic, transnasal cannulation of the intrasellar mass. On each occasion 4 to 6 ml of dark, partly clotted blood and necrotic fragments of adenoma were aspirated, with rapid improvement of vision. In one case pre-operative intractable hypotension responded poorly to large doses of corticosteroids and pressor drugs. The operative stress of this procedure is minimal and, followed by radiotherapy, it seems ideal in such cases.

SURGICAL TREATMENT OF THE CRANIOPHARYNGIOMAS

Considering the congenital origin and benign histological appearance of the craniopharyngiomas until fairly recently their surgical treatment has produced disappointing results. This is in part due to their adherence to, but not their infiltration into, surrounding vital structures but perhaps, even more, to the profound biochemical disturbances immediately following hypothalamic damage.

Before the introduction of corticosteroid therapy Love and Marshall (1950) quoted a mortality of 41 per cent following attempts at total extirpation of these lesions and Peyton, French and Baker (1955) stated 'the surgical treatment of craniopharyngiomas is highly unsatisfactory and survival ranges from a few months to a few years even with multiple operations and aspirations.' In 1968, Sutcliffe Kerr presented a survey of 41 cases spanning a period of 20 years. One-third had survived this period but only one-sixth had total removal of the tumour. In the second period of 10 years, of 11 cases, 10 had major surgery with five deaths. Three of the five survivors had complete excision of the tumour, the others had a partial removal. Such results which were probably somewhat better than average at the time, not unnaturally led to a trial of minimal surgery combined with high dose, megavoltage irradiation. McKissock and Ford (1966) reported 55 cases of craniopharyngioma subjected to major surgery of which only 12 remained alive, well and working at periods of one to over 10 years compared with 33 of 45 patients having minor surgery (cyst aspiration and, where indicated, ventricular drainage) plus radiotherapy. This approach was first described in 1961 by Kramer, McKissock and Concannon and 'further experience and late results' were provided by Kramer, Southard and Mansfield (1968).

A demonstration of the effects of this form of treatment is provided by the following case history and illustrations provided by Mr Julien Taylor.

CASE HISTORY
Youth B.B., now 22 years old, at the age of fourteen developed signs of increased intracranial pressure without visual loss. The cyst was aspirated and radiotherapy given in 1966 (Co 60 4000 rads, T.D. in 26 days with 6 x 6 cm fields). The cystograms are illustrated and the most recent films show a marked shrinkage of the cyst. The boy is very well, with normal vision and is now studying accountancy (Figures 6.2 to 6.8).

The combination of skilled, high voltage radiotherapy and minimal surgery seemed the best that could be offered in the treatment of craniopharyngiomas until Matson and Crigler (1960) described a remarkably successful series of 13 cases subjected to radical surgical excision. In a further report (Matson and Crigler, 1969), there was no operative mortality in 40 patients operated on primarily in their clinic. Thirty-six of these were thought by the surgeon to have had a total removal. An additional 17 cases had been operated on elsewhere in the first instance. Total excision was achieved in 10 of these with seven subtotal excisions and a post-operative mortality of five cases. The post-operative deaths occurred in attempts to remove tumours previously operated on in other clinics one or more times and all but one of these had also had radiotherapy. However, not all patients undergoing secondary operations ended badly as the last five such patients in this series have had successful secondary total excisions.

As with any other tumour, total eradication without unacceptable damage must be regarded as the ideal. Without repeating details of the long-term study of the subsequent development of these children, which are available in Matson's papers (1960, 1969), it can

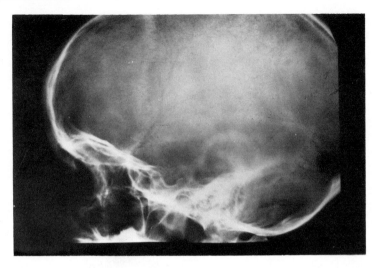

Figure 6.2. Plain film showing faint suprasellar calcification.

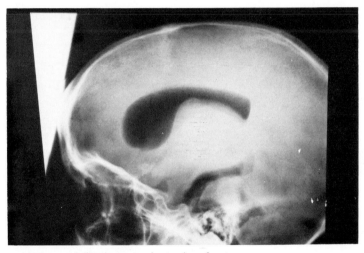

Figure 6.3. Air ventriculogram indicating upward extension of cyst.

be said that with the aid of substitution therapy, the majority of these patients lead fairly normal lives. There was an initial mortality of five, already mentioned, and a later mortality of eight. Of the 44 survivors, 38 were attending school or working normally, two were attending schools for the blind and there were also two well infants. Two children were invalids, both having been left with residual tumour tissue after secondary operations. Diabetes insipidus persists to some degree in most patients and, in general, when an extensive removal of tumour tissue from within the sella turcica is carried out, the surgeon must be prepared to treat his patient acutely as though hypophysectomised and chronically

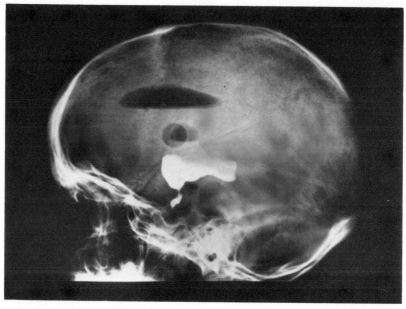

Figure 6.4. Film after aspiration of cyst and introduction of one ml of steripaque. The stalk running to the pituitary fossa represents the remainder of the craniopharyngeal canal.

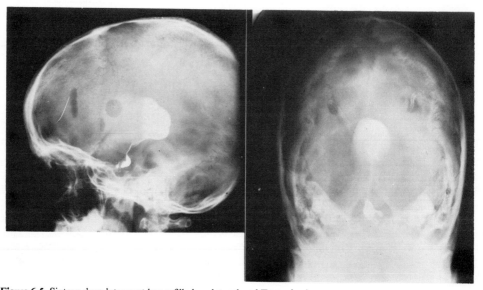

Figure 6.5. Sixteen days later cyst has refilled — lateral and Towne's views.

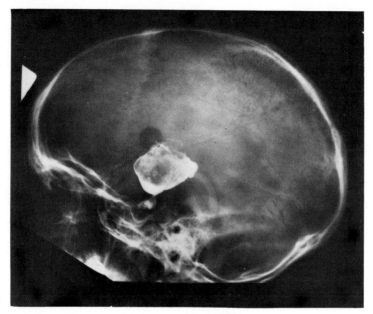

Figure 6.6. Six months later following further aspiration and DXT.

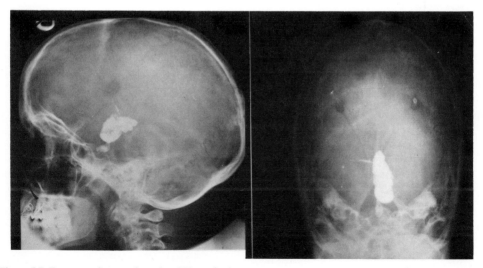

Figure 6.7. Four years later — lateral and Towne's views.

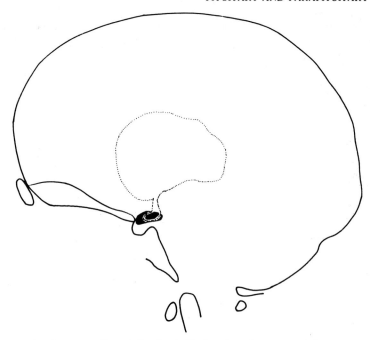

Figure 6.8. Diagram showing suprasellar calcification in black and maximum extent of cyst.

as having deficiency in antidiuretic hormone, thyroid, adrenal and gonad function, and impairment of normal growth. Most patients require some supplementary thyroid treatment but few were dependent upon cortisone, except in situations of stress.

There are two main reasons for the striking differences between the results of Matson and his followers and of those who preceded them. The first is technical, related to the use of corticosteroids and precise biochemical control on the one hand and the introduction of improved anaesthesia and operative magnification on the other. The second reason refers to a positive state of mind of the surgeon who now knows either vicariously or from his own experience that it is no longer justified to regard these lesions as being beyond the scope of surgery. The two factors fortify each other, as is particularly evident in the persistence required for the dissection of such lesions under visual magnification.

Corticosteroid therapy and water balance over the period of operation have been described earlier in this chapter. Pitressin is not used in the immediate post-operative period until urine output exceeds 150 ml/hour, but in any case output is balanced by an equal volume of appropriate intravenous fluid. Pitressin in oil or pitressin snuff are not indicated until the patient is well into the convalescent period.

Surgical Technique

A prime object of the neurosurgical anaesthetist is the reduction of brain volume, but in these cases dehydrating agents should not be employed for this purpose. There may well be difficulty with water balance without this additional factor. Late cases with hydrocephalus benefit from a previous shunting procedure. Transfrontal craniotomy, usually on the right side, extending to the midline and as low as possible is employed. It may be necessary with solid tumours to amputate the frontal pole to improve access which is otherwise much improved by emptying a cyst. The frontal lobe should be elevated by a self-retaining brain retractor so that the operator has both hands free. Sometimes removal of the tuberculum is indicated to improve access to a large, solid, probably calcified, intrasellar tumour.

Illumination and magnification are provided by either the operating microscope or by a good head lamp and magnifying spectacles. The dissection is described by Matson as follows '. . . with a firm grasp on the capsule either between the optic nerves, lateral to the chiasm, or immediately behind the chiasm exactly in the midline, to begin a meticulous mobilization of the tumour from surrounding structures. The tumour which has been dissected free should never be excised completely, but only to an extent of about one-half or less, so as to leave a good handle to hold on to and continue gradual delivery of the tumour, from wherever it goes, to the suprasellar region. The parts under the brain stem, in the Sylvian fissures, or protruding into the third ventricle usually come forward cleanly in this manner. The tumour is usually removed piecemeal. Occasionally, in the presence of a large cyst which can be emptied, the whole lesion may be removed intact. We have never sacrificed an optic nerve nor incised the chiasm'.

Whatever the radiological appearances may suggest, a transventricular approach is to be avoided, as serious hypothalamic damage by this route is inevitable. Dissection from below, as described, gives the best chance of success. Finally, despite the most painstaking dissection it is obvious that small pieces of tumour may be missed or indeed may have to be left deliberately and therefore recurrence is always possible, but even so results now available from a number of clinics confirm the advantages of the radical approach to this group of tumours.

Craniopharyngiomas in the Elderly

Although more than 50 per cent of craniopharyngiomas manifest themselves in children under 12 years, about one-third of cases have their first symptoms after the age of 40 and in a series of 160 patients, 14 were between the ages of 60 and 72. As was pointed out by Ross Russell and Pennybacker (1961), in adults there is much less tendency for the tumour to obstruct the flow of cerebrospinal fluid and the incidence of endocrine abnormality also falls sharply. Visual failure from chiasmal compression remains common and mental disturbance, a rare feature in young patients, becomes of increasing importance.

These cases most frequently present with disturbances of vision and as 40 per cent show no radiological abnormality of the sella or tumour calcification (Banna, 1973), their pre-operative diagnosis may be in some doubt. They are a lesser surgical problem as a rule than are the craniopharyngiomas of childhood. They are often smaller, affecting the chiasm rather than the foramina of Monro, and are more likely to be removed completely. Even if they are not completely excised their growth rate seems to be much less, as might be inferred from their age of presentation.

The Trans-sphenoidal Operation

In that small group of craniopharyngiomas, usually in the adult, which are intrasellar in origin and have not progressed to a significant suprasellar extension, trans-sphenoidal surgery has an important place. The technique has already been described and it is in such cases that it may be possible, with the aid of the microscope, to spare sufficient compressed pituitary tissue to the patient's subsequent advantage.

PARASELLAR TUMOURS

The approach to these tumours is determined by their location as indicated radiologically. Thus classical frontal craniotomy is appropriate for the meningiomas of the tuberculum sellae and those in the region of the anterior clinoid process. Gliomas of the optic nerve and chiasm are similarly approached, with unroofing of the orbit for complete removal when the operability of the intracranial portion of the tumour has been determined. Meningiomas of the sphenoidal ridge call for a more lateral, fronto-temporal craniotomy and the more posteriorly placed tumours, meningiomas of the posterior clinoid process, of the greater wing and of the clivus are dealt with through a temporal craniotomy. The transclival operation for meningioma and chordoma of the clivus has been described by Stevenson et al (1966) and by Decker and Malis (1970).

Usually the primary object in the operative treatment of the parasellar tumours is to relieve pressure on the optic nerves and chiasm. These structures, already suffering the effects of pressure, may be very sensitive to even the slightest further trauma at operation. The tumour is, therefore, gradually reduced in volume anteriorly or laterally, i.e. distal to important structures, until there remains a 'shell' of tumour tissue protecting the nerves and sometimes the internal carotid artery and its branches. With appropriate illumination and magnification the remaining portion of a meningioma, usually with gentle traction and a little at a time, separates readily but it is important to preserve small vessels running on the chiasm and to the hypothalamus (Dawson, 1958). With the exercise of caution such a removal in most cases is a fairly straightforward procedure, but situations do arise in which a decision must be made regarding subtotal removal and, very occasionally, the sacrifice of a damaged optic nerve trapped by tumour.

There are three circumstances in which it may be more prudent to leave a small piece of tumour rather than risk the serious consequences of persisting to the end. A meningioma may not only be firmly attached to the carotid artery, its bifurcation and its branches, it may grow around them and, indeed, as can sometimes be demonstrated angiographically, it may constrict and eventually occlude them. A patent bifurcation should not be endangered in an attempt to remove the last small piece of meningioma tissue and the risks to a contained carotid artery at the initial 'intracapsular' stage of tumour removal should also be borne in mind. Judgment should be similarly exercised when a large suprasellar tumour extends into and is adherent to the hypothalamus. A middle fossa meningioma may be attached medially to the wall of the cavernous sinus and may separate from below upwards until it can be detached at the clinoid process. Bleeding can then be controlled by gentle pressure on Gelfoam. Here also a small amount of tumour may have to be left.

A parasellar meningioma may spread in the region of the optic foramen as if it were en plaque and may strangle the optic nerve by forming a narrow ring around it. If the eye on that side is already blind there can be no objection to dividing the optic nerve and removing this extension of the tumour as there is always the fear of spread across the midline. If there is some worthwhile remaining vision, however, it is futile to attempt to preserve or to improve it by removing tumour tissue from around the nerve or growing into the canal. This part of the tumour should be ignored. Similar considerations apply when a piece of meningioma traps the optic nerve by passing under it near the foramen. The situation is particularly difficult when the tumour also involves the carotid artery. When there is reason to suspect such complexities it is probably justified to warn the patient before operation that he may lose the sight in a badly affected eye in order to preserve the vision in the good eye.

Optic Nerve Glioma

These tumours are usually very slow growing and predominantly affect children. The important distinction is between involvement of one optic nerve and involvement of the chiasm. A glioma of one optic nerve in the orbit causes painless proptosis with initially a central or paracentral scotoma. Extension backwards may produce radiologically evident enlargement of the optic foramen. This process may continue until the chiasm is involved and field defects occur in both eyes, but this is more likely to be the result of a primary chiasmal glioma when there may be enlargement of both foramina. Davis (1940) described bilateral involvement in nearly 50 per cent of his cases. Chiasmal tumours may grow to a large size and spread into the hypothalamus and third ventricle. If this can be demonstrated radiologically it should be regarded as a contra-indication to radical surgery, although some sort of ventricular drainage procedure and radiotherapy may be considered worthwhile.

In a case of primary unilateral optic nerve glioma as radical a removal as possible should be attempted. This is best achieved by frontal craniotomy and inspection of the intradural optic nerve and the chiasm. The dura is then stripped from the roof of the orbit which is removed together with the roof of the optic canal. The most favourable circumstance would be one in which it was possible to divide the optic nerve in front of the chiasm and behind the globe and to remove the tumour completely without removing the globe or interfering with the vision of the other eye at the chiasm. If the glioma had spread to the eyeball this would have to be removed subsequently by the ophthalmologist. When the chiasm is just involved an attempt at radical removal should be made if the visual fibres from the other eye are not put at risk, otherwise biopsy only is indicated. These patients should probably be given post-operative radiation but in such slow growing astrocytomas the results, and indeed the rationale, of this are not easy to determine. Thus Matson (1969) describes four patients with only biopsy or partial intracranial excision surviving 21, 17, 14 and 12 years. Tym (1961) recorded three patients in whom the tumour invaded the chiasm who were alive 15, 17 and 18 years later with useful vision. Following radical excision of an optic nerve glioma it would be reasonable to expect a permanent cure and radiotherapy would not be justified. However, Hoyt and Baghdassarian (1968) showed that even chiasmatic and hypothalamic involvement is compatible with long survival. They reviewed 36 patients, three to 41 years after presentation. Ten had died; one immediately after operation, four of hydrocephalus, three of sarcomatous degeneration of extracranial neurofibromas and two of other causes. By inference the remaining 26 were alive, although in 29 of the original 36 the tumour affected the chiasm and hypothalamus. They emphasise the good prognosis, not only for life but also of vision. It is against this background that various forms of treatment must be assessed. Four out of five of their cases with signs of hydrocephalus died despite cerebrospinal fluid shunting procedures and radiotherapy. These writers conclude that neither excision, other than for relief of proptosis, nor radiotherapy is justified.

In contrast to the benign optic nerve gliomas of childhood attention has been drawn by Hoyt et al (1973) to the rare malignant astrocytomas of the anterior visual pathways occurring usually in middle-aged males which are invasive and lethal neoplasms. Their report described five new cases and referred to 10 previously recorded cases and they came to the conclusion that malignant optic gliomas in adult life comprise a distinct clinical and pathological entity. The initial symptoms in this condition are monocular blurring of vision and retrobulbar pain simulating optic neuritis but very soon the pattern of visual loss indicates involvement of the chiasm and within five to six weeks the patient is completely blind. Death occurred in most cases in less than a year with signs of extending neurological involvement in the latter stages of the disease. The progressive changes in the fundal appearance are characteristic, vascular occlusion in the distal segment of the optic nerve producing venous stasis, oedema and ischaemic infarction of the optic disc. Post-mortem examination shows extensive involvement of the optic nerves, chiasm and tracts by vascular and partially necrotic tumour tissue which may also involve the hypothalamus and adjacent parts of the brain. In the orbit this tissue spreads through the meninges into the tissue surrounding the optic nerve and histologically it appears to be of glial origin and of a high malignancy.

The Empty Sella Syndrome

Primary examples of this condition, causing progressive visual impairment with headache and occasionally rhinorrhoea, are probably due to the formation of an arachnoid cyst in the sella through an unusually large diaphragmatic opening (Busch, 1951; Kaufman, 1968). The secondary type is a consequence of surgery for pituitary tumour, usually associated with irradiation. Here the optic nerves are distorted, perhaps with secondary ischaemic changes, by traction as the diaphragm descends into the sella. In these cases there is often firm adherence between the nerves and chiasm and the diaphragm. Typically, following visual improvement after surgery, deterioration occurs two or three years later (Colby and Kearns, 1962; Lee and Adams, 1968). This may, rightly or wrongly, be attributed to irradiation damage and air encephalography may help to decide. If doubt remains the chiasm should be inspected by transfrontal craniotomy.

In the primary condition it may not be difficult to free the chiasm and elevate it into its normal position by filling the sella with muscle, as described by Wood and Dogali (1975). But the firm adhesions of the secondary type may prevent this. Welch and Stears (1971) improved such a patient's vision by injecting normal saline through the diaphragm to relieve tension on the chiasm and maintained its new position by filling the sella with silicone sponge. Olson, Guiot and Derome (1972) recommend elevation of the diaphragm and optic structures by a trans-sphenoidal, microsurgical approach. If at the time of the initial excision of the adenoma there is rapid fall of the diaphragm into the sella cavity these authors pack the sella with bone fragments to prevent subsequent descent and traction. This has been their practice in over 200 pituitary adenomas since 1966 and in 1972 they had seen no new case of a symptomatic empty sella.

REFERENCES

Bakay, L. (1950) The results of 300 pituitary adenoma operations (Professor Herbert Olivecrona's series). *Journal of Neurosurgery*, **7**, 240.
Banna, M. (1973) Craniopharyngioma in adults. *Surgery and Neurology*, **1**, 202-204.
Bateman, G. H. (1963) Trans-sphenoidal hypophysectomy. *Proceedings of the Royal Society of Medicine*, **56**, 393.
Busch, W. (1951) Die Morphologie der Sella turcica und ihre Beziehungen zur Hypophyse. *Archiv für Pathologische Anatomie*, **320**, 437.
Colby, M. Y. Jr & Kearns, T. P. (1962) Radiation therapy of pituitary adenomas with associated visual impairment. *Proceedings of the Staff Meeting of the Mayo Clinic*, **37**, 15.
Davidoff, L. M. (1962) Symposium on pituitary tumours — IV. Discussion of papers. *Journal of Neurosurgery*, **19**, 22.
Davis, F. A. (1940) Primary tumours of the optic nerve. (A phenomenon of Recklinghausen's disease.) *Archives of Ophthalmology*, **23**, 735–821, 957–1022.
Dawson, B. H. (1958) The blood vessels of the human optic chiasma and their relation to those of the hypophysis and hypothalamus. *Brain*, **81**, 207–217.

Decker, R. E. & Malis, L. S. (1970) Surgical approaches to midline lesions at the base of the skull. A review. *Mount Sinai Journal of Medicine* (New York), **30**, 84.

Elkington, S. G. & McKissock, W. (1967) Pituitary adenomata: Results of combined surgery and radiotherapeutic treatment of 260 patients. *British Medical Journal*, **i**, 263.

Guiot, G. & Thibaut, B. (1959) L'extirpation des adenomes hypophysaires par voie trans-sphenoidale. *Neurochirurgie*, **1**, 133.

Hamlin, H. (1962) The case for trans-sphenoidal approach to hypophyseal tumours. *Journal of Neurosurgery*, **19**, 1000.

Hardy, J. (1969) *Clinical Neurosurgery*, p.16. Baltimore: Williams and Wilkins.

Hardy, J. (1971) Trans-sphenoidal hypophysectomy. *Journal of Neurosurgery*, **34**, 581.

Hardy, J. (1974) Trans-sphenoidal microsurgical removal of pituitary adenoma. In *Recent Progress in Neurological Surgery*, p.86. Amsterdam: Excerpta Medica.

Henderson, W. R. (1939) The pituitary adenomata: A follow-up study of the surgical results in 338 cases (Dr. Harvey Cushing's series). *British Journal of Surgery*, **26**, 811.

Hirsch, O. (1910) Endonasal method of removal of hypophyseal tumours. With report of two cases. *Journal of the American Medical Association*, **55**, 772.

Hirsch, O. (1956) Pituitary tumours. A borderland between cranial and trans-sphenoidal surgery. *New England*

Hirsch, O. (1959) Life-long cures and improvements after trans-sphenoidal operation of pituitary tumours. (Thirty-three patients followed for 20–37 years.) *Acta Ophthalmologica* (Kobenhavn), (Supplement), **56**, 60.

Horrax, G. (1958) Treatment of pituitary adenomas. *Archives of Neurology and Psychiatry* (Chicago), **79**, 1.

Horsley, V. (1906) On the technique of operation on the central nervous system. *British Medical Journal*, **ii**, 411.

Hoyt, W. F. & Bahdassarian, S. A. (1968) Optic glioma of childhood. Natural history and rationale of conservative management. *British Journal of Ophthalmology*, **53**, 793.

Hoyt, W. F., Meshel, L. G., Lessell, S., Schatz, N. J. & Suckling, R. D. (1973) Malignant optic glioma of adulthood. *Brain*, **96**, 121.

Ingraham, F. D. & Matson, D. D. (1954) *Neurosurgery in Infancy and Childhood*. Springfield, Illinois: Charles C. Thomas.

Jefferson, A. A. (1969) Chromophobe pituitary adenomata: The size of the suprasellar portion in relation to the safety of operation. *Journal of Neurology, Neurosurgery and Psychiatry*, **32**, 633.

Jefferson, G. (1940) Extrasellar extensions in pituitary adenomas. *Proceedings of the Royal Society of Medicine*, **33**, 433.

Jefferson, G. (1957) Sir Victor Horsley (1857-1916) Centenary Lecture. *British Medical Journal*, **i**, 903.

Kaufman, B. (1968) The "empty" sella turcica — a manifestation of the intra-sella subarachnoid space. *Radiology*, **90**, 931.

Kerr, A. S. (1968) Craniopharyngiomata. *Journal of Neurology, Neurosurgery and Psychiatry*, **31**, 646.

Kramer, S., McKissock, W. & Concannon, J. P. (1961) Craniopharyngiomas. Treatment by combined surgery and radiation therapy. *Journal of Neurosurgery*, **18**, 217.

Kramer, S., Southard, M. & Mansfield, C. M. (1968) Radiotherapy in the management of craniopharyngiomas. Further experience and late results. *American Journal of Roentgenology*, **103**, 44.

Lee, W. M. & Adams, J. E. (1968) The empty sella syndrome. *Journal of Neurosurgery*, **28**, 351.

Love, J. G. & Marshall, T. M. (1950) Craniopharyngiomas (pituitary adamantinomas). *Surgery, Gynaecology and Obstetrics*, **90**, 591.

Matson, D. D. & Crigler, J. F. Jr (1960) Radical treatment of craniopharyngiomas. *Annals of Surgery*, **152**, 699.

Matson, D. D. & Crigler, J. F. Jr (1969) Mangement of craniopharyngioma in childhoold. *Journal of Neurosurgery*, **30**, 377.

McKissock, W. & Ford, R. K. (1966) Results of treatment of the craniopharyngiomas. *Journal of Neurology, Neurosurgery and Psychiatry*, **29**, 475.

Olson, D. R., Guiot, G. & Derome, P. (1972) The symptomatic empty sella — prevention and correction via the trans-sphenoidal approach. *Journal of Neurosurgery*, **37**, 533.

Peyton, W. T., French, L. A. & Baker, A. B. (1955) Intracranial neoplasms. In *Clinical Neurology* (Ed.) Baker, A. B. 1st edition. New York: Hoebner.

Poppen, J. L. (1959) The temporal approach to tumours of the sella turcica in the presence of a prefixed chiasma. *Journal of Neurology, Neurosurgery and Psychiatry*, **22**, 79.

Poppen, J. L. (1963) Changing concepts in the treatment of pituitary adenomas. *Bulletin of the New York Academy of Medicine*, **39**, 21.

Ray, B. S. & Patterson, R. H. (1962) Surgical treatment of pituitary adenomas. *Journal of Neurosurgery*, **19**, 1.

Ross Russell, R. W. & Pennybacker, J. B. (1961) Craniopharyngioma in the elderly. *Journal of Neurology, Neurosurgery and Psychiatry*, **24**, 1.

Stevenson, G. C., Storey, R. J., Perkins, R. K. & Adams, J. E. (1966) A transcervical, transclival approach to the ventral surface of the brain stem for removal of a clivus chordoma. *Journal of Neurosurgery,* **24,** 544.

Tym, R. (1961) Piloid gliomas of the anterior optic pathways. *British Journal of Surgery,* **49,** 322.

Uihlein, A., Balfour, W. M. & Donovan, P. F. (1957) Acute haemorrhage into pituitary adenomas. *Journal of Neurosurgery,* **14,** 140.

Welch, K. & Stears, J. C. (1971) Chiasmapexy for the correction of traction of the optic nerves and chiasm associated with their descent into an empty sella turcica. *Journal of Neurosurgery,* **35,** 760.

Wood, J. H. & Dogali, M. (1975) Visual improvement after chiasmapexy for primary empty sella turcica. *Surgical Neurology,* **3,** 291.

Zervas, N. T. & Mendelson, G. (1975) Treatment of acute haemorrhage of pituitary tumours. *Lancet,* **i,** 604.

CHAPTER SEVEN

Radiotherapy of the Pituitary Gland

W. M. ROSS

In the majority of the disorders of the pituitary gland for which radiotherapy is given there is no malignancy – a benign adenoma produces either endocrine or pressure effects. It is well established that the endocrine function of such a gland is not appreciably depressed by the required doses of radiation, which are below those in the 'carcinocidal' range (Kelly et al, 1951). Furthermore there are, closely adjacent to the pituitary gland, a number of structures which are liable to suffer harmful changes following exposure to relatively small doses of irradiation. It is therefore interesting that for some sixty years radiotherapy has contributed to the management of patients with pituitary gland disorders, because for many of these years the apparatus used produced radiations of relatively low penetrating power with poor collimation, and assessment of the effects of treatment was entirely clinical. Thus Cushing's series of pituitary tumours reported by Henderson (1939) depended with respect to their response to radiotherapy on the use of low energy equipment of a type which would no longer be used for such patients. The beneficial results, with a relative absence of untoward side effects, were most encouraging. Kramer (1968) noted that most tumours of the pituitary or parapituitary tissues are histologically benign and yet respond well to radiation. Malignant tumours such as gliomas of the floor of the third ventricle or ectopic pinealomas occur rarely at this site, but can also be treated satisfactorily by irradiation.

The last twenty years have seen very rapid developments in the practice of medicine and surgery in relation to the pituitary gland. Reference is made elsewhere to improvements in diagnostic methods, in particular to contrast neuroradiology, and to radio-isotope scanning techniques. More accurate methods of endocrine diagnosis by assay of hormones and hormone releasing factors have also been introduced. Parallel to these advances radiotherapy techniques have improved, so that it is now possible to deliver the desired dose very accurately to a limited volume of tissue with less exposure of adjacent sensitive tissues. In addition, following treatment, hormone replacement substances are now available to counteract hormone deficiencies. It is not surprising, therefore, that in the modern practice of radiotherapy, using beams of radiation of high energy and good collimation, and with the recently developed assays of the several hormones produced by the pituitary gland, there has been little if any reduction in the use of radiotherapy. It seems appropriate to consider at this stage the continuing place of radiotherapy in the management of pituitary disorders.

PITUITARY DISORDERS IN WHICH RADIOTHERAPY IS USED

The two principal aspects of pituitary disorder which raise the question of radiation therapy are anatomical abnormalities of the pituitary gland and its environs and abnormalities of endocrine secretion by the gland. As the majority of pituitary disorders are not malignant such anatomical abnormalities are due to mechanical displacement of adjacent tissues rather than to neoplastic invasion and destruction. As we shall see, particularly at risk from irradiation are the bony walls of the sella, the hypothalamus and the floor of the third ventricle, the optic tract, chiasm and nerves, and the third, fourth and sixth cranial nerves as they pass alongside the sella in the wall of the cavernous sinus. Bloom (1973), however, considers that the optic chiasm appears to be relatively tolerant of irradiation. Either aspect of pituitary disorder, i.e. anatomical or endocrine, may be associated with changes in the relative proportions of the different types of normal anterior pituitary cells, namely basophil, eosinophil and chromophobe. It would appear that any one of these types of cells may be produced in excess, either spontaneously, or possibly in relation to a stimulus from the hypothalamic releasing factor mechanism. Such an excess of cells may produce a diffuse involvement of the greater part of the pituitary gland or an isolated nodule or adenoma. In either case the excess of cells of one particular type tends to impair the function of other cells of the pituitary gland by compression. Such depression of activity of otherwise normal pituitary cells may lead to a similar reduction of activity of the target cell or gland, as in hypothyroidism, or it may also stimulate production of the suprapituitary releasing factor with compensatory overgrowth of the affected normal cells, sometimes leading to secondary adenoma formation.

Of the anatomical effects, one of the earliest associated with minimal increase in the size of the sella is headache, probably due to stretching of the periosteum, although on occasion a very considerable enlargement of the sella is found in a patient who denies any headache. The other possibility is that the gland will enlarge upwards, with or without significant enlargement of the bony sella, elevating the diaphragma sellae, to which the optic chiasm is related. The resulting disturbance of vision has been described in Chapter 4. Upward extension of the tumour past the normal position of the diaphragma sellae will elevate the floor of the anterior part of the third ventricle and may lead to distortion or obstruction of the foramina of Munro and distension of the lateral ventricles.

In order to consider the place of radiotherapy, disorders of the pituitary gland are classified according to the clinical endocrine picture or syndrome presenting and this will be done in the following sections.

ACROMEGALY

Acromegaly is the syndrome resulting from the prolonged excessive secretion of growth hormone in patients past the age of fusion of the epiphyses and is characterised by excessive growth in bulk of bony and soft tissues. Important side effects include an increased morbidity and mortality from hypertension and left ventricular hypertrophy. A strong indication for treatment, therefore, is the reduced life expectancy of such patients. Wright et al (1970) showed that mortality is almost double that expected from a general population of similar structure, the increased deaths being due to cardiovascular or respiratory disease or to clinical diabetes. The disease varies very considerably in severity as evidenced by the magnitude and rapidity of the anatomical changes in the bones and soft tissues, and to some extent this is mirrored by the levels of growth hormone detectable in the peripheral blood. There can be little doubt that in some patients the disease does become 'burnt out' with a return to relatively low growth hormone figures, but in the majority there is, prior to any such 'burnt out' state, a period often measured in decades of progressive anatomical abnormality, continued hypertension and left heart strain. It can be shown that very real benefits accrue from treatment which leads to a return of the growth hormone to normal limits, i.e. preferably to not more than 5 ng/ml. Kramer (1968) noted that although radiotherapy often appears to be satisfactory in arresting acromegalic changes, in reversing the visual field and acuity changes and in controlling headache, growth hormone levels may not be reduced to normal and may continue to represent a danger to the patient's life. Despite this view he maintains that hypophysectomy is not indicated and that radiation therapy remains the treatment of choice.

The investigation of patients with acromegaly is outside the scope of this Chapter, but it is important to stress the need for exact determination of the position of the diaphragm by air encephalography, so that treatment can be accurately planned to include the whole of the affected pituitary tissue and to reduce to a minimum the risk to adjacent sensitive structures, particularly the optic chiasm.

The aim of treatment in acromegaly is to reduce the excessive secretion of growth hormone, if possible to within normal limits, as described above, and preferably without depressing the normal production of the other anterior lobe secretions. There is, however, little evidence that it is possible to achieve satisfactory depressions of growth hormone by radiotherapy without producing some degree of pan-hypopituitarism requiring replacement of other endocrine hormones, in particular TSH, ACTH and gonadotrophins.

Techniques of radiotherapy will be described later, but it is desirable here to consider the relative merits of the various forms of treatment available. External beam therapy using a linear accelerator generating x-rays at 4 to 10 MeV, enabling a high energy, finely collimated beam to be directed at the pituitary gland, with a satisfactory sharp cut-off outside the immediately desired treatment area, is the method of treatment most commonly used today. It has been repeatedly shown that doses between 4000 and 5000 rads given in four or five weeks in daily fractions produce a slow fall in growth hormone levels, which may not be maximal for up to four years (Roth, Gorden and Brace, 1970), with an acceptably low level of untoward complications involving the optic tract, chiasm and hypothalamus. There is evidence of diminished response when a lower dose is given but an increase in the dose beyond 5000 rads in five weeks does not appear to produce any significant improvement in results and is likely to lead to an increased incidence of adverse side effects. Aloia, Roginsky and Aichambeau (1974) described a small series of patients given 5500 rads, none of whom developed visual field defects. Although, usually, patients with field defects are not treated initially by external beam therapy, cases have been reported with visual field defects due to suprasellar extension which have improved following external beam therapy. Following such treatment there is little evidence of altered secretion of other anterior lobe hormones, and therefore little risk of hypoadrenalism, hypothyroidism or hypogonadism. Wright (1970) described a satisfactory clinical response in more than half his cases, although associated with hypopituitarism in about one-quarter. He stressed that there was little change in the growth hormone levels in the first six months after external irradiation but a significant reduction to half over the next 18 months. However, the fact that reduction in growth hormone levels is delayed, often for years, has led to some dissatisfaction with the use of external beam therapy alone, even when it is accepted that the ultimate levels of growth hormone some years after treatment may be reduced satisfactorily.

External beam therapy is at present, in most centres, the method of choice for the relatively mild acromegalic without evidence of rapid progression of the disease, without very high growth hormone levels and without any evidence of suprasellar extension or visual field defects. Even this statement may soon be questioned, when the effects of bromocriptine in producing temporary depression of growth hormone secretion are fully assessed. However, the slow response to x-ray treatment has led to a more detailed study of other methods of depressing the activity of the gland such as surgical hypophysectomy, cryosurgery, interstitial irradiation and heavy particle beam therapy. The latter method, requiring the availability of a synchrotron or similar apparatus, is limited to a very few centres. The other three methods cause a very high or complete degree of destruction of the affected tissues and while effective in controlling acromegaly invariably lead to pan-hypopituitarism.

Of the newer methods interstitial irradiation is the one which has been used most frequently by the implantation of one or more sources of radiation inside the pituitary gland. The isotopes first used were radon, which is no longer available, and gold which, though mainly a beta-ray emitter, has approximately a 10 per cent gamma emission. The latter is considerably more penetrating and may deliver an undesirably high dose to those tissues immediately adjacent to the sella. Finally yttrium, which is purely a beta-ray emitter, the electrons having a maximum range of approximately 1.1 cm in tissue, has been more in favour of recent years. Suitably accurate positioning of one to four yttrium rods of size and radioactivity especially calculated for the particular patient, enables the gland to be irradiated to a pre-determined minimum dose — the maximum dose near to the anatomical centre of the gland and in physical contact with the yttrium rods being almost infinitely high. Providing, therefore, that the exact dimensions of the sella are determined by tomography, together with the position of the diaphragma sellae and the optic nerves and chiasm from air encephalography, the dose to neighbouring structures can be controlled and the incidence of side effects reduced to a very low level. Following interstitial irradiation the growth hormone levels usually fall quite quickly, particularly during the first year, though a further fall may be evident for at least another year. This is often followed by improvement in the patient's symptoms and signs, although there is not necessarily a close correlation between the gross anatomical features and growth hormone levels. Very occasionally changes in the size of the digits and loosening of rings etc. may be apparent within a few days of the implant. Molinatti et al (1962) described improvement in all patients treated by implantation, with no evidence of subsequent relapse and a significant improvement in associated severe diabetes. He commented on the difficulty in deciding on the appropriate dose, the aim being to suppress the hyperactive tissue only.

It is not my purpose to comment on the surgical treatment of acromegaly except to say that following transfrontal craniotomy and partial removal of the gland to decompress the chiasm there was usually no change in the acromegalic state and as in the treatment of the chromophobe adenomas post-operative irradiation is indicated. In some centres surgical ablation of the pituitary gland at craniotomy has been completed by packing the fossa with wax impregnated with radioactive yttrium in the hope of destroying any surviving cells (Edelstyn, Gleadhill and Lyons, 1964).

Combined treatment

It is of course possible and often helpful to combine interstitial irradiation with external beam therapy. For example, a patient with a very large tumour which had been decompressed surgically followed by external beam therapy may have achieved only partial remission, which could be improved by yttrium implantation. In these circumstances it would almost certainly be unsafe to repeat the external beam therapy. Alternatively, after initial treatment by yttrium rods with only partial response, it may be possible to repeat the treatment or to supplement it by external beam therapy. In all cases where further treatment is being considered air encephalography should be repeated to ensure that the new position of the diaphragm is known, and that all abnormal tissue may be included in the radiation field. It is particularly important to recognise depression of the diaphragm as, if an yttrium implantation by the inferior route is planned, the depressed portion of the diaphragm may be so close to one of the implanted rods as to suffer an area of radio-necrosis leading to CSF rhinorrhoea. The other condition which it is important to exclude is the 'empty sella' syndrome which may follow radiotherapy, or occasionally occur spontaneously, and in which progressive visual deterioration is associated with marked depression of the diaphragma sellae and associated distortion of the optic chiasm. Progressive degenerative changes, particularly in the small vessels, sometimes follows irradiation and, if this is aggravated by anatomical distortion or mechanical pressure, complete ischaemia of the involved tissues may follow. The 'empty sella' syndrome is of course an absolute contraindication to further radiotherapy. Lee and Adams (1968) suggest that the cause may be arachnoiditis of the optic nerves and tracts and that the syndrome is more common after combined surgery and radiation than after either alone.

CUSHING'S SYNDROME

Cushing's syndrome, due to a pituitary or suprapituitary cause, is an indication for irradiating the pituitary gland to reduce ACTH levels and the consequent effects of excessive cortisone production by the adrenals. The natural history of patients with this syndrome is one of progressive disability associated with hypercortisolaemia causing obesity, osteoporosis and hypertension with a diminished expectation of life. Welbourne, Montgomery and Kennedy (1971) showed that 30 per cent of patients with Cushing's syndrome were dead within two years and 50 per cent within five years of diagnosis. A spontaneous improvement, possibly due to infarction of the pituitary gland, is rather more common in this condition than in acromegaly. The possibility of an autonomous adrenal cause (hyperplasia, adenoma or carcinoma) must be excluded, as no significant effect is to be expected from pituitary irradiation in such patients. Kramer insists that irradiation of the pituitary should be used as the primary form of treatment only where an adrenal tumour has been excluded and where there is no evidence of enlargement of the sella and hyperplasia of the adrenals.

The form of treatment almost invariably employed in these patients is that of external beam therapy using a high energy, well collimated linear accelerator or telecobalt beam and giving a dose of 4500 rads to the pituitary in four to four and a half weeks. It is advantageous to monitor any changes in the visual fields during and immediately after the treatment, because it has been reported that a transitory increase in the size of the gland and some initial deterioration in visual fields may occur. If mild this would indicate delay in further irradiation and if excessive or prolonged would be an indication for surgical decompression. Edmunds, Simpson and Meaking (1972) described their experience with 17 patients with pituitary driven Cushing's disease, over 12 years, treated with telecobalt radiation in whom the majority had a complete remission with no complications. Following treatment the plasma levels of cortisol and ACTH fall towards normal but the full effects of the treatment are often not apparent for at least a year and in this time it is often helpful to use aminoglutethimide and metyrapone to depress the secretion of ACTH. Following such irradiation of the pituitary in patients with Cushing's syndrome, replacement therapy in relation to other pituitary hormones is seldom necessary. In some patients in whom the disease has been so active and so prolonged that organic changes have developed in the adrenal glands, which do not resolve when the ACTH stimulus is removed, subsequent adrenalectomy may be indicated. Interstitial implantation of the pituitary for Cushing's syndrome has been advocated by some writers but is not frequently used. One series from the Hammersmith Hospital (Burke, 1973) indicated, perhaps not surprisingly, that the degree of response was dependent on the size of the gland. Of 31 patients with fossae of normal size 65 per cent showed complete remission, despite the fact that some 50 per cent of these patients had benign tumours rather than mere hyperplasia of the anterior lobe of the pituitary. Of 10 patients with doubtfully enlarged sellae, only five had complete remission, whereas of 14 patients with definitely enlarged sellae, of whom three-quarters had tumours, a remission was seen in only two, and it was concluded that the patients with large sellae require radiation to both the pituitary and to the adrenals. At least 50 per cent of the patients who had undergone implantation treatment required replacement therapy for partial or complete hypopituitarism.

NELSON'S SYNDROME

Following bilateral adrenalectomy for hyperplasia or tumour, a small proportion of patients have developed Nelson's syndrome, characterised by weakness, lethargy and progressive pigmentation of the skin, often to quite a dark brown colour. This is associated with hyperactivity of the ACTH-producing cells of the anterior pituitary, and presumably also of the MSH-producing cells, and there have been a number of such patients in whom external beam therapy to the pituitary gland has proved effective in controlling or leading to a reversal of the excessive pigmentation. There is a 10 per cent incidence of Nelson's syndrome in patients with Cushing's disease treated by adrenalectomy alone, but an almost negligible incidence in patients treated by irradiation of the pituitary followed by adrenalectomy. In these patients a dose of 4000 to 4500 rads in four to four-and-a-half weeks using an external beam from a linear accelerator is appropriate treatment.

CHROMOPHOBE ADENOMA

In this section reference will be made to those patients with pituitary abnormalities who do not fall readily into the categories already mentioned. Endocrine abnormalities tend to be most commonly deficiency of gonadotrophins, or prolactin, but often there may be no detectable endocrine abnormality and the presenting feature is headache with or without visual field disturbances, and an enlarged sella. Unless there is evidence of a visual field defect it is unlikely that surgery will be necessary, and therefore that histological proof of the type of the tumour will be available, but there appears to be a less complete correlation between histology and the endocrine effects of the tumour than was formerly thought to be the case. Again a profile of the endocrine secretions and an air encephalogram are necessary for a complete assessment.

Treatment Policy

In formulating a treatment policy for these patients, it should be remembered that most have no visual field defects and no evidence of suprasellar extension and that treatment with external beam therapy will usually be effective. Sheline, Boldrey and Phillips (1964) reported that most authors rely upon irradiation to control the growth of these adenomas but views vary on the necessity for preliminary decompression. There is evidence of an increased response following increased dosage and an optimal dosage would appear to be 4500 to 5000 rads over four-and-a-half to five weeks. In patients with a small visual field defect and no evidence on air encephalography of suprasellar extension, initial treatment by radiotherapy is often sufficient, leading to a slow improvement in the visual field defects over the next six to twelve months, but it is essential that during the period of treatment the visual fields are frequently checked for any deterioration. Chang and Pool (1967) reported that one-third of cases of chromophobe adenoma treated primarily by irradiation required surgical decompression and stated that up to 40 per cent of pituitary adenomas showed significant cyst formation which did not respond to irradiation without preliminary decompression. Hayes, Davis and Raventos (1971) considered that radiation alone was the treatment of choice except where there is rapid progression of visual loss. Ray and Patterson (1971) recommended that post-operative irradiation for chromophobe adenoma should be reserved for recurrences. Elkington and McKissock (1967) reported combined surgical and radiotherapeutic treatment of 260 patients and said that the indication for surgery was almost invariably impairment of vision, rarely enlargement of the adenoma due to haemorrhage and occasionally mental or other neurological symptoms supervening on an intracranial space-occupying lesion. Bloom's policy (1973) has generally been surgery combined with post-operative irradiation, though he admits that there was some selection in favour of a group receiving radiation alone, in that many early cases with small tumours had been included. On the other hand a few elderly advanced cases with longstanding poor vision, considered unsuitable for surgery, are to be found in the irradiation alone series. The survival rates at five years are identical but the combined treatment appears to give a rather better result, both as regards longer expectation of life and freedom from recurrence.

Henderson (1939) concluded that irradiation prevented or delayed post-operative recurrence and found no evidence of harmful effects from such treatment even after 15 years. Sheline, Boldrey and Phillips (1964) stated that only 16 per cent of his cases with chromophobe adenoma treated by surgery without radiation were without recurrence at the end of five years, whereas 82 per cent were free of recurrence after treatment by surgery and radiotherapy.

Late post-radiation changes

As indicated above there is little early change following irradiation but progressive changes in the visual field defects and the endocrine profile are to be expected over the next year or so and replacement therapy may become necessary, either as a temporary or a permanent measure. If, after initial improvement in the visual fields, there is subsequent visual deterioration a decision must be made as to whether this is due to a recurrence of the initial cause, i.e. the pituitary adenoma, or to late radiation effects such as fibrosis and endarteritis, or to the 'empty sella' syndrome already mentioned. It is likely to be necessary to repeat the air encephalogram and craniotomy may occasionally be necessary to elucidate the problem. In patients in whom a recurrence of residual tumour is confidently diagnosed, the question of further treatment arises; it is seldom, if ever, safe to repeat a course of external beam therapy because the risk of damage to adjacent tissue is very high indeed but the same risks do not apply to interstitial irradiation. In these circumstances a minimum dose of 50 000 rads within the pituitary gland would be indicated, as compared with a minimum 150 000 rads which is normally given to patients with acromegaly. Similarly in patients who have evidence of an invasive or malignant tumour, either on histological examination or from serial radiographs of the sella, the response to initial radiotherapy may be inadequate and further treatment by implantation may become indicated. Although it is difficult to be certain about the incidence of recurrence and late radiation effects these were both estimated, in our series, to be five per cent or less.

CRANIOPHARYNGIOMA

This congenital tumour presents with destructive and erosive features though histologically it has none of the characteristics of a malignant tumour. Although the majority occur in children a smaller number appear in adults of all ages and in them the prognosis is rather better. Craniopharyngioma is not a particularly radiosensitive lesion but there is long experience of at least some control of the condition by external beam radiotherapy and also of an improvement in the prognosis after surgery if deep x-ray therapy is then added. The tumour tends to recur after surgery, which can seldom be expected to be a complete excision because of the situation of the lesion. A method of management which has a considerable degree of favour and success is surgical exploration and removal of the bulk of the tumour, particularly any suprasellar extension, followed by radiotherapy to the residue. Kramer, Southard and Mansfield (1968) state that the results are particularly encouraging in children and recommend a definite place for radiation treatment of craniopharyngiomas following neurosurgery. As an alternative in the patients in whom the lesion is very largely a thin-walled cyst with little solid tumour present, aspiration of the cyst fluid and the insertion of a rather smaller volume of radioactive colloidal yttrium has been used effectively in some patients.

RADIOTHERAPY OF THE PITUITARY FOR OTHER CONDITIONS

Secondary Carcinoma

The sphenoid bone and the pituitary gland may be the site of secondary carcinoma, the two most common primary sites being the lung and the breast. These lesions are treated by the method appropriate to bone metastases from the particular site of the primary tumour, i.e. usually external beam radiotherapy combined with hormonal measures or cytotoxic chemotherapy. The dose of radiotherapy required is usually not in excess of 3000 rads and seldom leads to any deficiency of pituitary function in addition to that which the secondary tumour deposit has already caused.

Pituitary ablation for systemic disease

The induction of pan-hypopituitarism has been shown to produce beneficial effects in some patients with extensive metastatic carcinoma, particularly secondary to breast carcinoma, and to a lesser extent prostatic carcinoma or malignant melanoma, and also in some patients with advanced and progressive diabetic retinopathy. In these patients total ablation of the anterior pituitary gland is necessary and high dose techniques, usually using interstitial irradiation, are employed.

RADIOTHERAPY TECHNIQUES

External Beam Therapy

This is the method of radiotherapy most commonly employed in the irradiation of the pituitary gland. Historically beams of 'conventional' x-rays generated at energies from 150 to 500 kV, most commonly in the 250 to 300 kV range, have been employed in a technique using multiple small fields directed at the sella turcica. Modern techniques use beams of x-rays generated at energies in excess of 1 000 000 V, or of ionising particles, in this country usually electrons, though occasionally neutrons are available. The source usually employed is a linear accelerator rather than a telecobalt machine, because of the more satisfactory collimation which can be achieved and consequent reduction in the penumbra.

Treatment Planning

The fact that the pituitary gland is closely related to structures such as the optic nerves, chiasm and tracts, the hypothalamus and brain stem, which are rather more radiosensitive than the pituitary gland itself, makes it necessary for external beam therapy to be given by meticulous and sophisticated techniques. To this end a beam directed system with multiple small fields accurately arranged in relation to the pituitary gland is employed. The first essential is exact localisation of the pituitary gland relative to the skull, and delineation of its extremities, particularly of any suprasellar extension, and this is likely to require air encephalography. When this information is available a decision must be made as to the approximate field arrangement, usually of three fields, i.e. one through the vertex and one through each temporal region, the latter being 'wedged'. From the radiographs an exact plan of the skull in the plane of the three proposed fields is drawn to scale and the proposed fields are drawn in on the plan using ready prepared depth/dose curves. The dose distribution in the irradiated volume is calculated, often with the aid of a computer, so that an accurate estimation is gained of the distribution of radiation within the target volume and in the adjacent areas of high radiosensitivity, in which it is essential to keep the dose to a minimum (Figure 7.1).

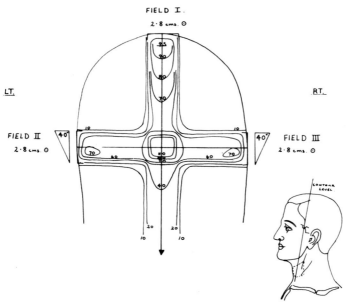

Figure 7.1. Field arrangement and dose distribution for external irradiation of pituitary adenoma.

When the plan of treatment as described above has been satisfactorily completed, an x-ray prescription is made out and arrangements are made for treatment to be given on the appropriate linear accelerator or similar apparatus. This necessitates an accurate and reproducible transfer of the size, position and angulation of each x-ray beam from the plan to the patient. Although the majority of radiotherapists employ a technique in which a beam direction shell is made specifically for the patient, it is possible with a cooperative patient to use skin marks related to known anatomical landmarks and so to obtain a similar accuracy of reproducibility for a course of treatment. There is little likelihood of any significant change in the shape or size of the head during treatment, but checks should be made at least once in the course of treatment that there has been no significant change in the soft tissues of the neck and shoulders when using the beam direction shell. Photographs of a typical beam direction shell on which are marked the points of entry and exit of the various x-ray beams are shown (Figure 7.2) and also the area of epilation which develops (Figure 7.3) at, or soon after, the end of the course of treatment. Meade (1973) described a stereotaxic method of x-ray treatment to the pituitary gland using six very small fields, generated by a linear accelerator, giving a tumour dose of 10 000 rads.

An alternative technique which is in favour in some centres is that of rotating the source of radiation around the patient during each course of treatment, either in a complete circle or in one or more arcs. This technique was developed in many centres when a telecobalt source apparatus was being installed and has the drawback of giving rather more radiation to the tissues close to the target volume than is the case with well-collimated linear accelerator beams. It also gives a rather symmetrical cylindrical volume of high dose, so that it is less appropriate in the case of target volumes which are not symmetrical and cylindrical.

Check films are taken at the end of the planning process on the simulator machine and also on the treatment machine, at the start of and during the course of treatment as required, particularly if there is suspicion of any change in the size of the lesion under treatment or of the skull itself. These films also provide a permanent record of the treatment which was delivered.

Dose

The dose of radiation from an external beam apparatus is normally given in five fractions per week over a number of weeks, usually at a weekly rate of about 1000 rads. The dose required to achieve effective hormonal suppression of a normal pituitary gland is almost certainly more than 10 000 rads (Kelly et al, 1951), a dose which is considerably in excess of that tolerated by the optic chiasm and associated structures. However, experience has shown that a lower dose to the pituitary gland is effective in suppressing the abnormal secretion and reducing the pressure effects of many of the diseases which have been described. To a considerable extent an increase in dose will lead to a greater effectiveness and it has been shown that doses of the order of 2500 rads are significantly less effective than those of 4500 rads. A consensus of opinion is that approximately 4500 rads in four and a half weeks from a linear accelerator beam is likely to be effective in controlling the majority of the disorders described above, without significant side-effects. Any further elevation of the dose will increase the incidence of complications unacceptably, and therefore a dose of approximately 4500 rads in four and a half weeks is modern practice for Cushing's disease, chromophobe adenoma and acromegaly. As has already been indicated a smaller dose is very often used for metastatic carcinoma, and in those few cases where there is evidence that the primary pituitary disorder is invasive it is necessary to deliver a higher dose, perhaps 5500 rads in five and a half weeks, accepting that a higher incidence of complications is unavoidable.

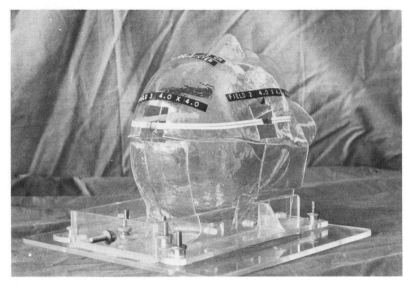

Figure 7.2. Beam direction shell.

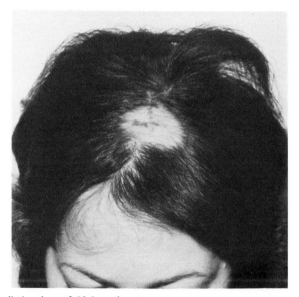

Figure 7.3. Area of depilation due to field through vertex.

Complications of external beam therapy

As already indicated the normal pituitary tissue is relatively radio-resistant and it is unlikely that treatment employing doses of the order already mentioned would lead to any degree of hypopituitarism requiring replacement therapy. Other late effects of radiotherapy are related to progressive changes in the fine vessels, particularly in the endothelium of arterioles, which appear as progressive endarteritis some years after treatment. This may lead to late ischaemic changes in the tissues supplied by the relevant vessels. In relation to treatment of the pituitary gland these are the optic chiasm and associated structures and the hypothalamus. The most common manifestation is a transient field defect, initially temporal and either unilateral or bilateral, often limited in extent and found by careful mapping of the visual fields. Occasionally, however this is more extensive and may progress to blindness. In such gross cases the changes are irreversible and are not amenable to any form of treatment. Effects on the hypothalamus may be manifest as a result of decreased secretion of antidiuretic hormone and consequent diabetes insipidus, which may develop relatively soon after treatment and may be transitory, or as a late and permanent phenomenon. In a very small number of patients changes in the cerebral vessels lead to serious mental disease and dementia. Peck and McGovern (1966) stress the danger of repeated courses of MXT and consider the deep white matter to be particularly radiosensitive. No indication for repeated courses of treatment was found.

In a small number of patients there may be a short-lived period of oedema of the irradiated tissues, especially during the first week or so of treatment, which may cause exacerbation of headache or temporary impairment of vision, usually in the form of concentric narrowing of the visual fields or occasionally of a temporal field defect. This form of reaction is temporary and can be diminished by reducing the daily dose of radiation or omitting the treatment for a few days until the phenomenon resolves. Correa and Lampe (1962) described improvement in the visual fields in patients with acromegaly and other pituitary adenomas treated with 250 kV x-rays and emphasised the relationship between dose and effect.

Intra-cavitary treatment

The frequency with which hypophysectomy was followed by recurrence of symptoms led to the practice in some centres of filling the empty sella with a wax material impregnated with radioactive yttrium to irradiate any remaining pituitary cells (Edelstyn, Gleadhill and Lyons, 1964). The author has no experience of this technique, which has not been used extensively. An alternative method was to swab out the sella with tissue fixative at the end of the excision.

Interstitial irradiation

The difficulty in delivering an adequate dose from external beam radiotherapy to the pituitary gland without risk of unacceptable complications, and the necessity in some patients to ablate the anterior pituitary gland completely, a procedure made possible when steroid replacement therapy became safe, has led to a variety of techniques to irradiate the gland by interstitial methods. Most have employed an inferior or anterior approach, using one or more sources of radioactive material introduced into the sella under radiographic control though in a small number of centres radioactive sources were introduced into the sella by craniotomy at the time of exploration of the pituitary gland. Initially an approach was made through the nasal cavity and sphenoidal air sinus (Forrest et al, 1959) but more commonly now an anterior approach through the ethmoid and spenoidal sinuses is used

(Joplin, 1965). To produce a satisfactory plan it is necessary to have exact dimensions of the sella, using tomograms in the AP and lateral planes, and air encephalography. Inactive yttrium rods of predetermined length are irradiated in the atomic pile to the necessary activity in millicuries, and introduced into the sella by the following technique. As the approach to the sella traverses the sphenoidal and ethmoidal air cells preliminary nasal toilet for 48 to 72 hours is necessary and prophylactic antibiotic cover starting on the day before the implant and continued for five days is usually prescribed. In addition, if nasal swabs taken during the two days prior to the implant indicate the presence of pathogenic organisms, other appropriate antibiotics are given. Endotracheal anaesthesia with pharyngeal packing is employed. Antero-posterior (Towne's view) and lateral radiographs to show the size and position of the sella are placed on the viewing box in the x-ray room in which the procedure is carried out, and the head is firmly supported in a perspex head clamp. The usual procedure, in which two rods are inserted one in either lateral half of the pituitary gland, is that which will now be described; if more than two rods are required the introductory process can be repeated. A 1-cm incision is made in the skin on the right side of the nose about 1 cm below and lateral to the nasion and the soft tissues divided until the nasal bone is exposed. A 3-mm hole is made in the nasal bone using a dental drill and a bone perforator is introduced and directed towards the sella turcica. The procedure is screened using an image intensifier and television monitor and frequent checks in planes at right angles to one another are made until the operator is satisfied that the bone perforator is directed correctly towards the right half of the sella turcica. The direction must be monitored to within about 1 mm before the anterior wall of the sphenoidal air sinus is perforated, as it is difficult to make corrections subsequently. The bone perforator is then advanced until it is in contact with the posterior wall of the sphenoidal air sinus which is the anterior wall of the sella. At this point the perforator is replaced by a cannula through which the remainder of the procedure is carried out. First a fine drill, 1·5 mm diameter with a centre point is introduced and the point is engaged in the anterior wall of the sella while final checks of direction are made in both planes. When the position is satisfactory the drill is advanced through the anterior wall making a 1.5 mm hole. The drill is replaced by a finer trocar and cannula which are advanced until the point of the trocar is touching the posterior wall of the sella. The sharp trocar is withdrawn and the yttrium rod introduced into the cannula and pushed forward by a threaded blunt-ended trocar. Under continuous television monitoring in the lateral position, the trocar is screwed forwards, using the blunt head as a pusher, until the yttrium rod is seen emerging from the end of the cannula into the sella. The trocar is advanced on the screw while the cannula is slowly withdrawn so that the yttrium rod is extruded into the pituitary gland until it can be seen to be separate from the cannula. Both inner and outer cannulae are then removed and the implant is complete for that particular rod. The above process of introduction is repeated as often as is necessary according to the initial prescription and final check radiographs are taken. Finally the skin incisions are sutured. Following the operation the patient is nursed supine for the remainder of the day until any postnasal bleeding has ceased.

Complications during the procedure

Haemorrhage from the ethmoidal air cells into the nose and pharynx is frequently rather copious and difficult to control during this procedure but almost invariably ceases spontaneously and does not demand any special care subsequently. Very rarely there is bleeding from inside the sella, or the leak of serous fluid from a cyst under tension inside the gland when the inner cannula is inserted and the sharp trocar removed for the insertion of the rod. The escape of fluid usually stops quite quickly but it is not considered wise in these circumstances to continue the implantation. Should significant bleeding continue from the sella a small piece of muscle may be inserted through the cannula to promote coagulation. Accurate positioning of the rods is sometimes prevented by movement of the rod after it has been extruded within the gland. This is associated with an unusually soft pituitary gland.

Post-operative complications

Some 48 to 72 hours following the implantation a degree of hypoadrenalism becomes apparent due to lack of ACTH unless the patient is on maintenance steroid replacement therapy. This may present with hypotension and malaise but more often is seen as an exacerbation of headache and some drowsiness which may not immediately be recognised as being associated with low levels of plasma cortisol. Depending on the radiation dose delivered to the pituitary gland, hypocortisolaemia and associated phenomena may or may not require permanent replacement therapy.

Diabetes insipidus, due to suppression of the hypothalamic antidiuretic hormone occurs in approximately one-third of patients, usually about a week after the implant. About 10 per cent of patients have this complication for a prolonged period, if not permanently, and may require treatment with pitressin, in the form of snuff, or chlorpropamide. In the majority of patients fortunately the complication is transitory and resolves spontaneously within about a month.

A more serious, but less frequent complication is cerebrospinal fluid rhinorrhoea. This is almost invariably associated with a small puncture of the diaphragm either due to the fact that the diaphragm itself is positioned rather low in the sella, or it is due to one of the rods being positioned higher than intended with a consequent, localised, very high dose area on the diaphragm. Wright described CSF rhinorrhoea in 15 per cent and local infection in 12 per cent of cases. Such an occurrence is obviously a possible source of meningitis by an ascending infection, and immediate antibiotic cover is indicated. The patient should also be nursed in the sitting position and have daily lumbar punctures. Very often this is sufficient to allow the fistula to heal, but if these measures are not successful the hole in the anterior wall of the sella must be plugged. Joplin (1965) has described a plug suitable for this purpose.

Doses from interstitial implants

For total ablation of the pituitary gland in the treatment of systemic disease such as progressive diabetic retinopathy or widespread metastatic breast carcinoma, a minimum dose of 300 000 rads is delivered within the pituitary gland. For acromegaly the author's present policy is to deliver a minimum dose of 150 000 rads, and on the rare occasions when pituitary adenomas are implanted, a minimum dose of 50 000 rads is indicated.

REFERENCES

Aloia, J. F., Roginsky, M. S. & Aichambeau, J. O. (1974) Pituitary irradiation in acromegaly. *American Journal of the Medical Sciences,* **267,** 81.
Bloom, H. J. G. (1973) Radiotherapy of pituitary tumours. In *Pituitary Tumours* (Ed.) Jenkins, John S. London: Butterworths.
Burke, C. W. (1973) Cushing's disease treated by pituitary implant. *Clinical Science,* **44,** 5.
Chang, C. H. & Pool, J. L. (1967) The radiotherapy of pituitary chromophobe adenomas: an evaluation of indications, techniques and results. *Radiology,* **89,** 1005.
Correa, J. N. & Lampe, I. (1962) Radiation treatment of pituitary adenomas. *Journal of Neurosurgery,* **19,** 626.
Edelstyn, G. A., Gleadhill, C. A. & Lyons, A. R. (1964) Attempted total hypophysectomy in advanced breast cancer. *British Journal of Surgery,* **51,** 32.

Edmonds, M. W., Simpson, W. J. K. & Meakin, J. W. (1972) External irradiation of pituitary for Cushing's disease. *Canadian Medical Association Journal,* **107,** 860.

Elkington, S. G. & McKissock, W. (1967) Pituitary adenoma — results of combined surgical and radiotherapeutic treatment. *British Medical Journal,* **i,** 263.

Forrest, A. P. M., Blair, D. W., Brown, D. A. P., Stewart, H. J., Sandeson, A. T., Harrington, R. W., Valentine, J. M. & Carter, P. T. (1959) Radioactive implantation of the pituitary. *British Journal of Surgery,* **47,** 61.

Fraser, T. R. & Wright, A. D. (1968) Treatment of acromegaly and Cushing's disease by Y90 implant. *Clinical Endocrinology,* **2,** 78.

Hayes, T. P., Davis, R. A. & Raventos, A. (1971) The treatment of pituitary chromophobe adenomas. *Radiology,* **98,** 149.

Henderson, W. R. (1939) The pituitary adenoma — a follow up study of surgical results in 338 cases. *British Journal of Surgery,* **26,** 811.

Jenkins, J. S., Ash, S. & Bloom, H. J. G. (1972) Endocrine function after external irradiation in patients with secreting and non-secreting pituitary tumours. *Quarterly Journal of Medicine,* **41,** 57.

Joplin, G. F. (1965) *Therapeutic Pituitary Ablation by Needle Implantation.* PhD thesis, London.

Kelly, K. H., Feldsted, E., Brown, R. E., Ortega, P., Bierman, H. R., Low-Beer, B. V. & Shrimkin, M. B. (1951) Irradiation of normal human hypophysis in malignancy. *Journal of the National Cancer Institute,* **11,** 967.

Kramer, S. (1968) The value of radiation therapy for pituitary and para-pituitary tumours. *Canadian Medical Association Journal,* **99,** 1120.

Kramer, S., Southard, M. & Mansfield, C. M. (1968) Radiotherapy in the management of craniopharyngiomas. *American Journal of Roentgenology,* **103,** 44.

Lee, W. M. & Adams, J. E. (1968). The empty sella syndrome. *Journal of Neurosurgery,* **28,** 351.

Mead, K. W. (1973) A radiotherapeutic technique for pituitary adenoma. *Australasian Radiology,* **17,** 250.

Molinatti, G. M., Massana, F., Olivetti, M., Pizzini, A. & Giuliani, G. (1962) Implantation of Y90 in sella turcica in cases of acromegaly. *Journal of Clinical Endocrinology and Metabolism,* **22,** 599.

Peck, F. C. & McGovern, E. R. (1966) Radiation necrosis of the brain in acromegaly. *Journal of Neurosurgery,* **25,** 536.

Ray, B. S. & Patterson, R. H. (1971) Surgical experience with chromophobe adenomas of pituitary gland. *Journal of Neurosurgery,* **34,** 276.

Roth, J., Gorden, P. & Brace, K. (1970) Efficacy of conventional pituitary irradiation in acromegaly. *New England Journal of Medicine,* **282,** 1385.

Sheline, G. E. (1971) Untreated and recurrent chromophobe adenomas of the pituitary. *American Journal of Roentgenology,* **112,** 768.

Sheline, G. E., Boldrey, E. B. & Phillips, T. L. (1964) Chromophobe adenomas of pituitary gland. *American Journal of Roentgenology,* **92,** 160.

Welbourn, R. B., Montgomery, D. A. D. & Kennedy, T. L. (1971) The natural history of treated Cushing's syndrome. *British Journal of Surgery,* **58,** 1.

Wright, A. D., Hill, D. M., Lowy, C. & Fraser, T. R. (1970) Mortality in acromegaly. *Quarterly Journal of Medicine,* **19,** 1.

Index

Note: Page numbers in *italics* indicate illustrations.

213